Oxford Specialist Handbooks published and forthcoming

General Oxford Specialist Handbooks
A Resuscitation Room Guide
Addiction Medicine
Perioperative Medicine,
Second Edition
Post-Operative Complications,
Second edition

Oxford Specialist Handbooks in Anaesthesia
Cardiac Anaesthesia
General Thoracic Anaesthesia
Neuroanaesthesia
Obstetric Anaesthesia
Paediatric Anaesthesia
Regional Anaesthesia, Stimulation and Ultrasound Techniques

Oxford Specialist Handbooks in Cardiology
Adult Congenital Heart Disease
Cardiac Catheterization and Coronary Intervention
Echocardiography
Heart Disease in Pregnancy
Fetal Cardiology
Heart Failure
Hypertension
Inherited Cardiac Disease
Nuclear Cardiology
Pacemakers and ICDs

Oxford Specialist Handbooks in Critical Care
Advanced Respiratory Critical Care

Oxford Specialist Handbooks in End of Life Care
End of Life Care in Cardiology
End of Life Care in Dementia
End of Life Care in Nephrology
End of Life Care in Respiratory Disease
End of Life Care in the Intensive Care Unit

Oxford Specialist Handbooks in Neurology
Epilepsy
Parkinson's Disease and Other Movement Disorders
Stroke Medicine

Oxford Specialist Handbooks in Paediatrics
Paediatric Endocrinology and Diabetes
Paediatric Dermatology
Paediatric Gastroenterology, Hepatology, and Nutrition
Paediatric Haematology and Oncology
Paediatric Nephrology
Paediatric Neurology
Paediatric Radiology
Paediatric Respiratory Medicine

Oxford Specialist Handbooks in Psychiatry
Child and Adolescent Psychiatry
Old Age Psychiatry

Oxford Specialist Handbooks in Radiology
Interventional Radiology
Musculoskeletal Imaging

Oxford Specialist Handbooks in Surgery
Cardiothoracic Surgery
Hand Surgery
Hepato-pancreatobiliary Surgery ·
Oral Maxillo Facial Surgery
Neurosurgery
Operative Surgery, Second Edition
Otolaryngology and Head and Neck Surgery
Plastic and Reconstructive Surgery
Surgical Oncology
Urological Surgery
Vascular Surgery

Oxford Specialist Handbooks in Cardiology
Heart Disease in Pregnancy

Edited by

Dawn L. Adamson

Consultant Interventional and Obstetric Cardiologist
University Hospital of Coventry and Warwickshire, UK

Mandish K. Dhanjal

Consultant Obstetrician and Gynaecologist,
Queen Charlotte's and Chelsea Hospital
Imperial College Health Care NHS Trust, London, UK

Catherine Nelson-Piercy

Consultant Obstetric Physician, St Thomas' Hospital,
Guys & St Thomas' Foundation Trust, Professor of
Obstetric Medicine, King's College, London, UK

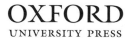

OXFORD
UNIVERSITY PRESS

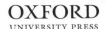

OXFORD
UNIVERSITY PRESS

Great Clarendon Street, Oxford OX2 6DP

Oxford University Press is a department of the University of Oxford.
It furthers the University's objective of excellence in research, scholarship,
and education by publishing worldwide in

Oxford New York

Auckland Cape Town Dar es Salaam Hong Kong Karachi
Kuala Lumpur Madrid Melbourne Mexico City Nairobi
New Delhi Shanghai Taipei Toronto

With offices in

Argentina Austria Brazil Chile Czech Republic France Greece
Guatemala Hungary Italy Japan Poland Portugal Singapore
South Korea Switzerland Thailand Turkey Ukraine Vietnam

Oxford is a registered trade mark of Oxford University Press
in the UK and in certain other countries

Published in the United States
by Oxford University Press Inc., New York

British Library Cataloguing in Publication Data
Data available

Library of Congress Cataloging-in-Publication-Data
Data available

Typeset by Glyph International, Bangalore, India
Printed in China
on acid-free paper through
Asia Pacific Offset

ISBN 978–0–19–957430–8

10 9 8 7 6 5 4 3 2 1

Foreword

Most health care professionals have doubts and anxieties when faced with a pregnant woman with heart disease. They need clear guidance and this book offers many of the answers and is essential reading for anyone who has an interested in this challenging but very satisfying area of medicine. It is also a mine of information to have by ones side as a reference text. In particular it deals thoroughly with normal pregnancy and the alterations in all things clinical including physical examination and investigations that occur in a normal pregnancy and puts these changes in the context of the normal altered physiology of pregnancy. The text is accessible to both cardiologists and non-cardiologist alike as each section summarises the cardiological features of the condition under discussion before embarking on its effect on pregnancy and the way that the problem should be dealt with to achieve a good outcome. Very sensibly there is an emphasis on how to anticipate trouble and put plans of action in place before problems develop. It also, at many points, makes it clear that in many situations where in the past Caesarean section has been thought to be the answer to problems with delivery in women with heart disease vaginal delivery is safe and often preferable. This book covers all aspects and runs from how to avoid pregnancy with detailed advice about contraception in the context of coincident heart disease, and advice before pregnancy for those a wanting to go ahead to assisted reproduction in women with heart disease . On the way it deals clearly with the management of well established but potentially dangerous cardiac conditions which are stable before and handling unexpected emergency situations. The common areas and problems e.g. dealing with oral and parenteral anticoagulants, managing blood pressure and rhythm disturbances are dealt with in detail but less common but important areas such as acute coronary syndromes in pregnancy are also dealt with thoroughly. There is also a very helpful section on the pharmacology of pregnancy.

The importance of truly multi-disciplinary approach to managing women with heart disease in pregnancy and the puerperium is stressed throughout. There is no other text I know of that takes on this difficult subject and deals with it so thoroughly and in such a practical manner.

Professor Roger Hall
Professor of Clinical Cardiology,
University of East Anglia, Norwich

and

Visiting Professor of Clinical Cardiology,
Imperial College,
London, UK

Preface

Heart disease is the commonest cause of maternal death in the UK. The woman presenting with cardiac disease in pregnancy, whether established or of new onset, often provokes fear and uncertainty in her carers. A multidisciplinary approach with the appropriate involvement of specialist cardiologists, obstetricians with training and experience in the management of high risk pregnancies and obstetric anaesthetists comfortable with the management of women with cardiac disease is essential. Expertise in the management of heart disease in pregnancy allows correct stratification of women into high and low risk and therefore facilitates normalisation of many women as well as optimisation of high dependency care required for those women at risk of severe complications.

This handbook is intended as a practical, easy-to-use reference to guide the clinician through the important issues to consider when caring for women with heart disease in pregnancy. For the obstetrician basic cardiological principles and investigations are explained and for the cardiologist ready reference chapters covering the unfamiliar territory of normal antenatal care, assisted conception and contraception are included. The Oxford Handbook style with clear diagrams and illustrations helps the reader of any discipline quickly access essential tips for the management of this challenging group of women.

DA
MKD
CNP

Acknowledgements

The authors would like to thank the following:

Drs Paul Clift and Sara Thorne for use of images from the *Oxford Specialist Handbook of Adult Congenital Heart Disease*.

The Department of Cardiac Investigations, University Hospital of Coventry and Warwickshire for help in obtaining the echo images.

Dr Richard Wellings and Dr Anna Herrey for supplying the MRI images and Dr Nigel Williams for his nuclear medicine image.

Dedications

Dawn Adamson

To "my boys", my husband Simon for putting up with me permanently attached to my lap top and to Ollie, for his constant offer of help; even if it was in the form of pressing the delete button when you least needed it with chocolate covered fingers! Thank you

Mandish K. Dhanjal

To Deqa

Contents

Contributors

Dr Anna Herrey
Specialist Registrar in Cardiology
University College London
London, UK

Dr Nishat Siddique
Specialist Registrar in Cardiology
Worchester Royal Hospital
Worcester, UK

Dr Vinnie Sodhi
Consultant in Obstetric
Anaesthesia
Queen Charlotte's and Chelsea
Hospital
London, UK

Dr Sara Thorne
Consultant Cardiologist
Queen Elizabeth Medical Centre
Edgbaston, Birmingham, UK

Abbreviations

ABG	arterial blood gas
ACE	angiotensin enzyme
aCL	anticardiolipin antibodies
ACS	acute coronary syndromes
ADH	antidiuretic hormone
AF	atrial fibrillation
AICD	automatic implantable cardiac defibrillator
ALP	alkaline phosphatase
ALT	alanine transaminase
APCR	activated protein C resistance
APS	antiphospholipid syndrome
APTT	activated partial thromboplastin time
AR	aortic regurgitation
ARB	angiotensin receptor blockers
ARDS	adult respiratory distress syndrome
ARM	artificial rupture of membranes
ART	assisted reproductive technologies
AS	aortic stenosis
ASD	atrial septal defect
ASH	asymmetrical septal hypertrophy
AST	aspartate aminotranferase
AT	antithrombin
AV	atrio-ventricular
BBB	bundle branch blood
BC	blood cultures
BMI	body mass index
BMS	bare metal stents
BP	blood pressure
bpm	beats per minute
CABG	coronary artery bypass grafting
CCU	coronary care unit
CEMACH	Confidential Enquiry into Maternal and Child Deaths
CHB	congenital heart block
CHD	congenital heart disease
CK/CKMB	creatine kinase/creatine kinase MB
CMRI	cardiac magnetic resonance imaging

CNI	calcineurin inhibitor
CNS	central nervous system
CO	cardiac output
COC	combined oral contraceptive pill
CS	caesarean section
CSE	combined spinal and epidural
CT	computed tomography
CTG	cardiotocograph
CTPA	computed tomography pulmonary angiogram
CVA	cerebrovascular accident
CVP	central venous pressure
CXR	chest x-ray
DAPT	dual anti-platelet therapy
DCM	Dilated cardiomyopathy
DES	drug eluting stents
DSE	dobutamine stress echocardiography
DVT	deep vein thrombosis
ECG	electrocardiogram
EDD	estimated date of delivery
EPS	electrophysiological studies
EROA	effective regurgitant orifice area
ETT	exercise tolerance testing
FBC	full blood count
FFP	fresh frozen plasma
FGR	fetal growth restriction
FVL	Factor V Leiden
GA	general anaesthesia
GIFT	gamete intrafallopian transfer
GFR	glomerular filtration rate
GnRH	gonadotrophin releasing hormone
GTN	glyceryl trinatrate
GTT	glucose tolerance test
HB	haemoglobin
hCG	human chorionic gonadotrophin
HCM	hypertrophic cardiomyopathy
HELLP	haemolysis, elevated liver enzymes, low platelets
HES	hydroxyethylstarch
HD	heart disease
HDL	high density lipoprotein
HFEA	Human Fertility and Embryology Authority

HIT	heparin induced thrombocytopenia
HOCM	hypertrophic obstructive cardiomyopthy
HR	heart rate
HS	heart sound
ICSI	intra-cytoplasmic sperm insemination
IE	infective endocarditis
IHD	ischaemic heart disease
INR	international normalised ratio
IOL	induction of labour
ISR	in stent-restenosis
ITU	intensive care unit
IUCD	intrauterine contraceptive devices
IUD	intrauterine device
IUI	in-utero insemination
IUS	intrauterine system
IVDU	intravenous drug use
IVC	inferior vena cava
IVF	in-vitro fertilisation
IVIG	intravenous immunoglobulin
IVSd	interventricular septum in diastole
JVP	Jugular venous pressure
LA	lupus anticoagulant
LA	left atrium
LBBB	left bundle branch block
LFT	liver function test
LMWH	Low molecular weight heparin
LNG-IUS	levonorgestrel intra-uterine system
LSE	left sternal edge
LVED	left ventricular end-diastolic
LVH	left ventricular hypertrophy
LVIDd	left ventricular internal dimension in diastole
LVIDs	left ventricular internal dimension in systole
LVOT	left ventricular outflow tract
MAPCA	major aortopulmonary collateral arteries
MC&S	microscopy, culture & sensitivity
MCV	mean corpuscular volume
MI	myocardial infarction
MMF	mycophenolate mofetil
MR	mitral regurgitation
MS	mitral stenosis

MSU	midstream urine
NSTEMI	non ST elevation myocardial infarction
NT	nuchal translucency
NTD	neural tube defects
NYHA	New York Heart Association
OHSS	ovarian hyperstimulation syndrome
OR	operating room
PA	pulmonary artery
PASP	pulmonary artery systolic pressures
PBMV	percutaneous balloon mitral valvuloplasty
PCI	percutaneous coronary intervention
PCR	protein creatinine ratio
PDA	patent ductus arteriosus
PE	pulmonary embolism
PET	pre-eclampsia toxaemia
PFO	patent foramen ovale
PGD	preimplantation genetic diagnosis
PHT	pulmonary hypertension
PIH	pregnancy-induced hypertension
PND	paroxysmal nocturnal dyspnoea
POP	progesterone-only pill
PPC	pre-pregnancy counselling
PPCI	primary percutaneous coronary angioplasty
PPCM	Peripartum cardiomyopathy
PPH	post partum haemorrhage
PPM	permanent pacemaker
PR	pulmonary regurgitation
PT	pro-thrombin time
PTT	partial thromboplastin time
PVR	pulmonary vascular resistance
PWd	posterior Wall in diastole
RA	regional anaesthesia
RA	right atrium
RAP	right atrial pressure
RBBB	right bundle branch block
RCOG	Royal College of Obstetricians and Gynaecologists
RDS	respiratory distress syndrome
RFA	radiofrequency ablation
RR	respiratory rate
rtPA	recombinant tissue plasminogen activator

RV	right ventricle
RVOTT	right ventricular outflow tract
SADS	sudden adult death syndrome
SLE	systemic lupus erythematosus
SOB	shortness of breath
SR	sinus rhythm
STEMI ST	elevation myocardial infarction
SVC	superior vena cava
SVR	systemic vascular resistance
SVT	supraventicular tacycardia
TCPC	total cavopulmonary connection
TENS	transcutaneous electrical nerve stimulation
TFT	thyroid function test
TGA	complete transposition of the great arteries
THR	target heart rate
TOE	transoesophageal echocardiogram
ToF	Tetralogy of Fallot
TR	tricuspid regurgitation
TSH	thyroid stimulating hormone
TTN	transient tachypnoea of newborn
UA	unstable angina
U&E	urea & electrolytes
UFH	unfractionated heparin
UH	unfractionated heparin
UPSI	unprotected sexual intercourse
USS	ultrasound scan
UTI	urinary tract infection
VDRL/TPHA	vene real disease research laboratory/treponema pallidum haemagglutination assay
VQ	ventilation-perfusion
VSD	ventricular septal defects
VTE	venous thrombo-embolism
WCC	white cell count
WPW	Wolff–Parkinson White syndrome
ZIFT	zygote intrafallopian transfer

1

Physiological changes in pregnancy

Introduction

The physiological adaptation to pregnancy causes significant changes in the cardiovascular system to allow the women to manage the increased metabolic requirements of the growing fetus.

Whilst women with normal cardiac structure and function can adapt well, women with cardiac disease may decompensate which can lead to significant complications in pregnancy and even result in fetal and maternal death.

Changes in the cardiovascular system are significant and occur early in the first trimester and as such, pregnancy may be the time when previously undiagnosed conditions become unmasked as a result of the reduced cardiac reserve.

The increase in work required by the heart is due to:
• growing fetus with increasing oxygen consumption
• enlarging uterus and breasts requiring greater oxygen demand
• increase in work by mother due to 10–14 kg weight gain
• placental bed acting like an arterio-venous fistula.

Physiological changes in the antenatal period

The physiological changes affect pre-load, intrinsic cardiac contraction, and the after-load.

Circulating blood volume

Cardiac preload is increased due to the increase in circulating volume which occurs from 6 weeks' gestation and plateaus by the end of the second trimester at a level 50–70% above the non-pregnant state.

Red cell mass also increases but only by 40% thus there is greater proportional increase in volume compared to red cell mass, leading to a relative haemodilution, the so called "physiological anaemia of pregnancy".

As a result of this blood volume increase, left ventricular end-diastolic (LVED) volume is increased which can be noticed on echocardiogram from 10 weeks' gestation. There is also a corresponding increase in atrial and right ventricular chamber dimensions, discussed further in Chapter 3.

This increase in blood volume creates particular problems for women with dilated cardiomyopathy and obstructive outflow lesions such as mitral stenosis or pulmonary hypertension.

Systemic and pulmonary vascular resistance

Systemic vascular resistance (SVR) is the resistance of all the peripheral vasculature in the systemic circulation, and this should not be confused with pulmonary vascular resistance (PVR), which is the resistance only in the pulmonary circulation.

SVR is measured by looking at the change in pressure across the systemic circulation from beginning to end and dividing it by the cardiac output:

$$SVR = \frac{(Mean\ arterial\ pressure - Mean\ venous\ pressure)}{Cardiac\ output\ (CO)}$$

The afterload is the force against which the cardiac muscle has to contract and typically is reduced in pregnancy due to the fall in SVR. This reduction in resistance occurs from the 5th week of pregnancy and usually reaches its nadir between 20 and 32 weeks of gestation. After 32 weeks, the SVR rises again until term by which it has exceeded its pregnancy level.

The reduction in SVR is due to a combination of increased circulating vasodilators, namely prostacyclin (PGI_2) and to the diversion of blood into the low impedance uteroplacental circulation.

There is significant increase in blood flow in the early stages of pregnancy; however, this is countered by a decrease in PVR, resulting in no net changes in pulmonary artery pressure.

Blood flow

The reduction in SVR results in increased flow to different anatomical beds and resulting physiological changes. Renal blood flow increases to 60–80% above pre-pregnancy levels and peaks in the third trimester. This change coincides with a 50% increase in glomerular filtration rate (GFR), which is why normal blood levels of creatinine in pregnancy are reduced (see Chapter 3).

Blood flow to hands and feet are increased, hence women have warm erythematous extremeties.

Nasal blood flow to the mucosa is also increased and women often complain of nasal congestion or stuffiness. Nose bleeds are also more common in pregnancy.

Blood flow to the breasts is increased and may cause painful breast engorgement.

Stroke volume and cardiac output

Stroke volume is the volume of blood expelled from the ventricle with each beat and is approximately 70mls in a healthy adult male. It is a major determinant of cardiac output (CO) as CO is the product of stroke volume and heart rate (HR), both of which are increased during pregnancy.

CO increases by approximately 30–50% reaching a peak at the end of the second trimester. The majority of CO increase is as a result of increase in stroke volume, though HR does contribute. HR is particularly important at the end of pregnancy, as the increase in stroke volume plateaus however the HR continues to rise.

Women who are unable to increase their CO, or who require elevated filling pressures to do so, may end up developing cardiac failure during pregnancy. Women with fixed COs in the form of stenotic valve lesions, are at risk of maternal and fetal compromise.

Heart rate

The increase in HR peaks in the late second or early third trimester and is usually 10–20 beats above pre-pregnancy levels, although there is a wide variation, and it is not uncommon to see women towards the end of their pregnancy with a sinus tachycardia.

Oxygen consumption

Maternal peak oxygen consumption can increase by 20–30% at term as a result of both the increase in maternal and fetal tissue mass as well as the increase in cardiac and respiratory work. The increase in myocardial oxygen consumption may therefore trigger ischaemia in women with significant coronary disease.

Table 1.1 Haemodynamic changes during pregnancy and the puerperium

	Pregnancy	Peripartum	Post-partum
Blood volume	↑	↑	↓
Systemic vascular resistance	↓	↑	↑
Stroke volume	↑	↑	↓
Cardiac output	↑	↑	↓
Heart rate	↑	↑	↓
Blood pressure	↓	↑	↑

Reproduced with permission from Lefoy and Adamson (2007) Heart Rhythm Disorders. In: Oakley and Warnes, eds., *Heart Disease in Pregnancy*. Wiley–Blackwell.

Metabolism
A normal pregnant woman can gain 10–14 kg throughout her pregnancy so this should be remembered when interpreting daily weight management in the management of heart failure.

The weight gain of pregnancy is usually distributed with approximately 2kg in the first trimester (though a weight reduction is not unusual in women with significant morning sickness or hyperemesis), 5 kg in the second and the remaining 5 kg distributed throughout the third.

A sharp rise in weight at the end of the pregnancy may reflect the fluid retention of pre-eclampsia.

Physiological changes in the peripartum period

The first stage of labour involves uterine contractions and they contribute to haemodynamic changes in two ways. Firstly, the uterine contractions can "squeeze" blood into the circulating volume and increase it by as much as 500 mls, the so called "autotransfusion" phenomenon. Secondly, the pain associated with uterine contractions leads to increases in circulating catecholamines with resulting increases in heart rate, blood pressure, and cardiac output.

In total, cardiac output in labour increases by approximately 10% and immediately after delivery, cardiac output can increase to a total of 80% above pre-pregnancy values due to a combination of autotransfusion and the sudden relief of inferior vena caval compression (see Figure 1.1). CO returns to pre-labour levels at about 60 min post delivery.

These haemodynamic changes can be influenced by pain relief and anaesthesia during pregnancy and are discussed further in Chapter 26.

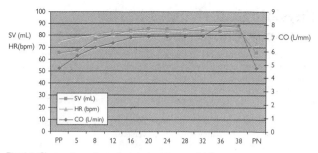

Fig. 1.1 Changes in cardiac output during labour and delivery.
Data from Robson *et al.* (1987) Cardiac output during labour. *BMJ* **295**, 1169–72.

Physiological changes in the post-partum period

The majority of haemodynamic changes will have returned to pre-pregnancy values by 3 months; however in some women full resolution may take as long as 6 months.

- *Blood volume*: Decreases by 10% 3 days post delivery.
- *Hb levels:* Increase steadily over the first 2 weeks post-partum then stabilize.
- *Blood pressure:* Falls initially and then increases day 3–7 postnatal. Returns to pre-pregnancy levels by 6 weeks.
- *SVR:* Increases over the first 2 weeks post-partum to 30% above delivery values.
- *HR:* Returns to baseline over first 2 weeks post-partum.
- *CO:* This increases by as much as 80% in the first HOUR post delivery but then continues to fall over the next 24 weeks post delivery.

Conclusion

Physiological changes in pregnancy are significant and occur as early as the first trimester to accommodate the growing uteroplacental unit and the fetus. Whilst they are well understood in the normal pregnant woman, it may not always be possible to predict how an individual with structural heart disease will tolerate such a magnitude of change. Understanding such changes, however, is important when looking after women with heart disease in order to possibly predict and be able to recognise complications as they occur.

The normal cardiac examination in pregnancy

Normal examination in pregnancy

The haemodynamic changes associated with pregnancy may be easily mis-interpreted as abnormal. This chapter describes the normal findings in pregnancy, and some pathological signs are also described.

General appearance

Firstly, observe the patient from the end of the bed – an obvious but often neglected place to start.

- **Respiratory rate (RR)** – normal is 12–20/min. Tachypnoea occurs when the RR > 22/min. During the later stages of pregnancy the gravid uterus increases pressure on the diaphragm and can lead to breathlessness. Women may also experience breathlessness at any stage of pregnancy probably related to the increase in minute ventilation.
- **Peripheral oedema** – increased blood volume and decreased venous return due to compression of the inferior vena cava from the gravid uterus, commonly cause peripheral oedema. This can mimic signs of right heart failure. If associated with hypertension and proteinuria oedema may herald pre-eclampsia and warrants urgent referral to the obstetrician.
- **Varicose veins** – these occur due to the increased circulating blood volume and vena-caval compression due to the gravid uterus.
- **Eye signs** – observe for exophthalmos or other signs of thyroid disease, anaemia, etc.

Pulse

Rate

- **Tachycardia** – the increased cardiac output and decreased peripheral resistance in pregnancy commonly creates a relative tachycardia. In the non-pregnant woman, the resting heart rate (HR) should be between 60–80 beats per minute (bpm). It is common for the pregnant woman to have a resting heart rate of around 90 bpm.
- **Bradycardia** – this is extremely rare and a HR of <50 bpm in a pregnant woman necessitates an ECG to rule out a brady-arrythmia and a medical review is recommended.

Rhythm

- Sinus rhythm should prevail in pregnancy but it is extremely common to develop ectopic beats (supra-ventricular and ventricular).
- Do not confuse an irregular pulse with AF as this may be SR with frequent ectopic beats – get an ECG to establish the precise rhythm.

Character

- **Bounding pulse** – this is a large-volume pulse, seen commonly in high cardiac output states such as pregnancy but also occurs with sepsis.

Blood pressure

How to measure BP in pregnancy

1. Ensure the patient is seated/lying comfortably at 45 degrees.
2. Apply the correctly sized blood pressure cuff to the right upper arm with the inflation bag over the brachial artery – a cuff that is too small will overestimate the BP.
3. Inflate the cuff until the radial pulse is no longer palpable.
4. Place the diaphragm of the stethoscope over the brachial artery just below the cuff.
5. Gradually reduce the pressure in the cuff a couple of mm of Hg at a time.
6. The first sound heard corresponds to the **systolic BP** and is known as the **1st Korotkoff phase**.
7. In non-pregnant patients, the pressure is decreased further until the sound disappears. This is the **diastolic pressure** and is known as the **5th Korotkoff phase**.
8. In pregnancy the 5th phase of the Korotkoff sounds is also taken as the diastolic pressure since the point where the sounds become muffled, known as the **4th Korotkoff phase** is not reliably reproducible.

BP drops early in the first trimester as there is a decrease in peripheral vascular resistance. It continues to drop gradually until 22–24 week's gestation and thereafter rises to pre-pregnancy levels by full term (see Chapter 1)

Jugular venous pressure (JVP)

- There is a direct connection between the internal jugular vein and the right atrium.
- The column of blood in the internal jugular vein acts as a surrogate marker of right atrial pressure.
- Outside pregnancy, elevated JVP (above 3–4 cm above the sternal angle) occurs frequently in heart failure, cardiac tamponade, constrictive pericarditis, and superior vena caval obstruction.
- Elevated JVP commonly occurs in late pregnancy due to increased circulating blood volume and compression of the vena cava by the gravid uterus.

Measuring the JVP

1. Position the patient at 45°.
2. The JVP is measured as the vertical distance from the sternal notch and the top of the venous column.
3. To differentiate between an artery and venous pulsation, gently compress the pulsatile vessel – the vein should stop pulsating but an artery will not.

Normal JVP is usually <3 cm but may be raised in the later stages of pregnancy.

Apex

A prominent, thrusting, non-displaced apical impulse due to the hyperdynamic state of pregnancy is common.

Heart sounds

- The 1st heart sound occurs due to the closure of the mitral and tricuspid valves.
- The 2nd heart sound is due to the closure of the aortic and pulmonary valves.
- During pregnancy, the hyperdynamic state causes **loud 1st and 2nd heart sounds.**
- The **3rd Heart sound** appears during early diastole and occurs after the 2nd heart sound. This creates a sound similar to a 'gallop' and is often described as a 'gallop rhythm'. This is a normal finding in children, young adults and pregnant women.
- The 4th heart sound occurs before the 1st heart sound, in late diastole and is always pathological.

Murmurs

Murmurs are heard due to turbulent flow.

During pregnancy, due to the high velocity of blood flow into slightly dilated cardiac chambers, turbulence occurs and systolic murmurs are common:

- Ejection systolic murmur audible in over 90% of pregnant women
  - It may be heard all over the precordium and even radiate to the neck and back
- Markers of a murmur that is more likely to be pathological are
  - Additional features, e.g. thrill, abnormal pulse character
  - Very loud systolic murmur
  - Known normal examination previously
  - **There should never be any diastolic murmurs and their presence is always pathological**
- Cervical venous hum – heard best over right upper sternal border due to increased venous return
- Mammary soufflé – continuous murmur due to increased mammary blood flow
- A loud second heart sound and a systolic murmur may mimic the signs of an atrial septal defect or pulmonary hypertension.

Investigations in pregnancy

Introduction

Investigation of the pregnant woman can be challenging for a number of reasons. Interpretation of results can be complex as physiological changes affect normal values, whilst some blood tests used to make diagnoses outside of pregnancy may be positive in the normal pregnancy. Some investigations are difficult to carry out due to the woman's physical condition whilst with others there may be fetal safety concerns.

This chapter aims to give a comprehensive overview of common investigations that may be required in the pregnant woman and discusses their use in pregnancy, any safety concerns to be considered, and any challenges in interpretation of the results.

General bedside/clinic investigations

Urine analysis

This cheap and simple test is essential in the routine investigation and management of a pregnant woman **(see Table 3.1):**

- Protein – if ≥ 1+ exclude urinary tract infection by sending MSU. If persistent proteinuria or hypertension check protein creatinine ratio (PCR) or 24 hour urinary protein collection to diagnose pre-eclampsia
- Blood – Commonly seen in urinary tract infections – but always check if suspecting infective endocarditis
- Leucocytes – if positive then send MSU for MC&S as urinary tract infections are more common in pregnancy
- Glucose – Pregnancy is a physiological state of relative glucose intolerance and insulin resistance, especially in the third trimester. This and the increase in glomerular filtration rate (GFR) means glycosuria is not uncommon and will frequently be ≥ 1.

Protein:creatinine ratio

Due to the difficulty in collection and unreliability of 24 hour urine collections, many units are now moving to spot urine protein:creatine ratios (PCRs). Normal is <30 mg/mmol and equates to approximately 0.3g/24 hours proteinuria. It therefore provides a useful screen for pre-eclampsia (see Chapter 15).

Table 3.1 Normal renal parameters in the pregnant and non-pregnant woman

	Non-Pregnant	Pregnant
Urea mmol/l	4.5–6	2.5–4
Creatinine μmol/l	60–105	40–80
Creatinine clearance mL/min	85–120	110–180
Urinary protein mg/24 hours	<150	150–300
Urinary glucose mg/24 hours	20–100 mg	10 mg–10 g/24 hours

Haematology blood tests

Normal haematological changes in pregnancy (See Table 3.2):

Relative anaemia – Hb 11–14g/dl

In pregnancy, the haematocrit (red cell mass) increases by 20–30% alongside a proportionally larger rise in plasma volume of 40–50%, thereby creating a relative anaemia. Physiological haemo-dilution peaks at 30 weeks of pregnancy and varies between individuals. It is more marked in multiple pregnancies.

Increased leukocytosis (WCC 6–16/mm³)

WCC and neutrophils increase in pregnancy and may rise further during labour. Corticosteroids given intramuscularly in large doses to induce fetal lung maturation will also cause a temporary leukocytosis. Do not rely solely on the WCC to diagnose an infection: check urine for leucocytes, nitrites, perform blood cultures if temperature > 38°C, look for signs and symptoms in both the pregnant woman and the fetus.

Abnormal haematological values in pregnancy

Anaemia – Hb < 10.5g/dL, HCT < 30%. This is usually due to either:

- **Iron-deficiency** which will lead to low iron levels, hypochromic, microcytic cells, low mean corpuscular volume (MCV) and an increased iron-binding capacity
- **Vitamin B$_{12}$/folate deficiency** which produces large cells and a high MCV
- Haemolytic anaemia is due to consumption of red blood cells and this leads to an increased reticulocyte count.

Table 3.2 Normal haematological parameters in the pregnant and non-pregnant woman

	Non-pregnant	Pregnant
Haemoglobin (Hb) g/dL	12–16	10.5–14
Haematocrit	36–48	30–36
White Cell Count (WCC) X 10⁹/L	4–10	6–16
Platelets X 10⁹/L	130–300	130–300
D-dimer	500	>500
INR	0.8–1.2	0.8–1.2

Coagulation blood tests

Normal coagulation

Clot formation occurs as a consequence of the clotting cascade (Figure 3.1). This is composed of two pathways – intrinsic and extrinsic. Each pathway consists of sequential steps involving clotting factors that eventually form a thrombus. Each factor is given a number.

The partial thromboplastin time (PTT) is a measure of the intrinsic pathway and is usually 23–37 sec and is used in monitoring the effects of unfractionated heparin therapy.

The pro-thrombin time (PT) measures the extrinsic pathway and is 11–12 sec. The international normalised ratio (INR) is 0.8–1.2 and is used to measure the anti-coagulant effects of warfarin.

Pregnancy is termed a 'hyper-coagulable' state. During pregnancy certain clotting factors (factors I, V, VII, VIII, IX, X, XIII) are increased leading to a higher risk of venous thrombosis. Due to the physiological changes in pregnancy, some of the tests for thrombophilia cannot be interpreted when the woman is pregnant.

D-dimer levels in pregnancy

D-dimers are released from thrombus and high levels are used to assess the probability of a venous thrombosis. Pregnancy as well as several other conditions, e.g. malignancy and sepsis, cause abnormally high D-dimer levels, which renders this test unhelpful in these settings.

Thrombophilia

The role of thrombophilias in venous thromboembolism is discussed in detail in Chapter 16. Here we will concentrate on the effect of pregnancy on the interpretation of the results.

Factor V Leiden

This occurs due to a mutation in factor V which results in resistance to activated protein C. Genotyping for this and the prothrombin 20210 gene mutation will not be affected by pregnancy but an activated protein C resistance is found in approximately 40% of pregnancies.

Protein C and protein S deficiency

These are endogenous anticoagulants that inhibit the coagulation cascade. Deficiency leads to an increased risk of thrombosis. Protein S levels fall in pregnancy so it is not possible to make a diagnosis of protein S deficiency in pregnancy.

Antithrombin (AT) deficiency

AT controls the coagulation cascade and deficiency leads to increased thrombogenesis. Whilst deficiency is rare in the general population, there is a 32–51% recurrence risk for thrombosis. Levels are unaffected by pregnancy but reduced in acute thrombosis.

Antiphospholipid antibodies

Anticardiolipin antibodies (aCL) and lupus anticoagulant (LA) are subsets of antiphospholipid antibodies and the combination of either of these with characteristic clinical features is known as antiphospholipid syndrome (APS). A diagnosis of APS requires 2 or more positive readings for LA +/or aCL at least 12 weeks apart plus one of the diagnostic criteria.

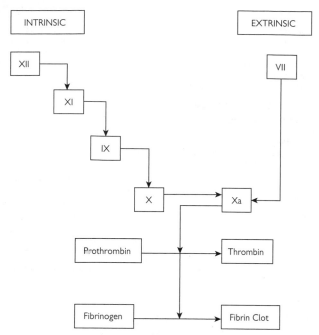

Fig. 3.1 The simplified coagulation cascade.

Renal function tests (see Table 3.1)

The increased plasma volume and decreased peripheral vascular resistance in pregnancy increases blood flow to the kidneys. Glomerular filtration rate (GFR) in pregnancy increases by 50%. Likewise, endogenous creatinine clearance is raised.

- Beware of the pregnant woman with a creatinine > 80µmol/l as this is likely to reflect renal impairment.

Liver enzymes (see Table 3.3)

In pregnancy the liver increases production of several substances:

- Lipids and cholesterol
- Clotting factors
- Increased alkaline phosphatase; this is released from the placenta as well as the liver and therefore should be raised in a normal pregnancy.

(*Note* – high levels of progesterone in pregnancy may cause delayed emptying of the gall bladder – therefore the risk of gallstones increases.)

Table 3.3 Normal liver enzymes and lipid tests for the pregnant and non-pregnant woman

	Non-Pregnant	Pregnant
Alanine transaminase (ALT) U/l	0–40	6–32
Aspartate aminotranferase (AST) U/l	7–40	10–30
Alkaline Phosphatase (ALP)	20–145	↑ 3–4 times normal value
Total cholesterol mmol/l	<5 mmol/L	↑ 40%
Total lipids mmol/l		↑ 40–60%
Triglycerides		↑ 200–300%

Thyroid function tests

TFTs change throughout pregnancy and it is important to examine the pregnant woman for signs and symptoms of thyroid disease before reaching a diagnosis.

It is thought that during the first trimester human chorionic gonadotrophin (hCG) stimulates the thyroid stimulating hormone (TSH) receptor and causes a rise in free T4 (FT4) which is biologically active and a fall in TSH. This effect is exaggerated in hyperemesis gravidarum.

Total T4 and T3 (which includes bound and free T4 and T3) increase during pregnancy and by the second trimester are 1.5 times higher than pre-pregnant levels. Serum FT4 and FT3 gradually decrease during pregnancy.

Table 3.4 Normal thyroid function tests during the different trimesters

	Non-preg	1st trimester	2nd trimester	3rd trimester
TSH mU/l	0.35–6.0	0.2–3.5	0.2–3.5	0.2–3.5
FT₃ pmol/l	3.5–7.7	3–5.7	2.8–4.2	2.4–4.1
FT₄ pmol/l	9–23	11.1–22.9	8.1–16.7	8.5–14.4

Reproduced from Cotzias C, Wong S, Taylor E, Seed P, Girling J (2008) A study to establish gestation-specific reference intervals for thyroid function tests in normal singleton pregnancy. *Eur J Obstet Gynecol Reprod Biol* **137**, 61–6. With permission from Elsevier.

Cardiac blood tests

Troponin: This is not raised in pregnancy and therefore can be used as a diagnostic tool to detect myocardial injury in the same way as when used in the non-pregnant woman (see Chapter 4)

CK levels in the normal pregnant woman are lower than the non pregnant woman. CK has been shown to rise during labour due to an increase in the muscle isoenzyme.

Normal levels of CK

Men	5–100 IU/L
Women	10–70 IU/L
Pregnancy	5–40 IU/L

ECG

The following findings are commonly seen in normal pregnancies:
- Sinus tachycardia
- 15° left axis deviation due to diaphragmatic elevation
- T-wave changes – commonly t wave inversion III and aVF
- Non-specific ST changes, e.g. depression
- Supra-ventricular and ventricular ectopic beats
- Small Q waves.

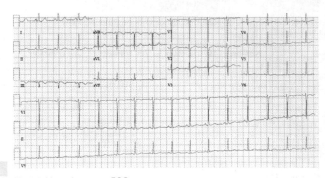

Fig. 3.2 Normal pregnant ECG.

Non-invasive cardiac investigations

Holter monitoring

This provides ambulatory measurements of heart rate, variability, and rhythm. Leads are attached to a small box which the patient wears attached to a belt for between 1–7 days. Holter monitors can either be worn to record all heart beats, e.g. 24 or 48 hour Holter or can be designed to monitor the heart continually but only record abnormalities in rate or rhythm. The choice of monitor depends upon the question being asked and the frequency of the 'palpitation' or arrhythmia you are trying to document.

Indications in pregnancy
- Palpitations
- Syncope and pre-syncope.

It is crucial the patient completes an 'event' diary which is compared with the recording in order to see if their symptoms correlate to an arrhythmia. As will be discussed in Chapter 8, many normal women have asymptomatic short runs of arrhythmia when monitored and these should not be treated unless thought to be dangerous.

Exercise tolerance testing (ETT)

This can be useful test in pregnancy as it is non-invasive and no radiation is involved, however, there is an increased false positive rate in non-pregnant women, and tests may be inconclusive due to fatigue.

Indications
- Used to objectively assess a woman's functional capacity.
- Diagnostic tool for ischaemic heart disease.
- Investigation of suspected exercise-induced arrhythmias.

Procedure
- Patients walk on a treadmill which has pre-set levels of speed and incline every 3 minutes. During the test they have regular BP monitoring and continuous ECG recording.
- The full Bruce protocol requires patients to exercise until 85% of the target heart rate (THR) is achieved (220 minus age for men, 210 minus age for women). Each stage lasts 3 minutes and there are 5 exercise stages.
- It may not be physically possible or safe to perform a full Bruce protocol ETT on a pregnant woman in the late stages of pregnancy but they may be able to exercise at a lower work load which starts off slower and with no incline (modified Bruce protocol).
- Normally, if patients are on a beta-blocker, then this is stopped 48 hours prior to the test as it may blunt the heart rate response. However, if you are aiming to assess the safety of a woman in pregnancy with known IHD, then it may be useful to continue it and see if she is ischaemic under her normal conditions.

Termination of test
- THR reached
- Patient complains of
  - Breathlessness
  - Chest pain
  - Pre-syncope/syncope
  - Fatigue
- Drop in BP or failure to rise with exercise
- Excessively high BP (> 220 mmHg)
- ST depression (> 2 mm)
- Frequent ventricular ectopics/VT
- Atrial arrythmis (but not ectopics)
- New BBB i.e. arrhythmias or AV block.

Normal contraindications to exercise testing

- Unstable angina.
- Pre-existing severe coronary artery disease (severe left main stem or equivalent disease).
- Uncontrolled hypertension (>220 mmHg systolic, > 120 mmHg diastolic).
- Decompensated heart failure.
- Aortic dissection.
- Severe Aortic stenosis.
- Underlying ECG abnormality where the ECG cannot be interpreted, e.g. left bundle branch block, LVH with 'strain pattern' (t wave inversion in lateral chest and limb leads). This applies only if looking for ischaemic change.
- Physical disability.

Contraindications to exercise testing in the pregnant woman
- Recent vaginal bleeding
- Placenta praevia
- Pre-eclampsia
- Symphyseal-pubic dysfunction/pelvic girdle dysfunction

Positive Test
- Failure of BP or HR to rise with exercise
- Typical anginal symptoms during exercise
- ST depression: ≥ 2 mm
- ST elevation*
- Ventricular arrhythmias*
- ST depression at low work-load, persisting into the recovery period*

*Consider urgent coronary angiography

Echocardiography

This is one of the most useful investigations as it is non-invasive and provides valuable information about cardiac structure and function in order to assess:

- cardiac dimensions
- left and right ventricular function
- valve anatomy and function
- intra-cardiac thrombus – either on valves or intra-mural
- infective endocarditis – **beware** – transthoracic echocardiogram (TTE) does not exclude this and a transoesophageal echo may be required
- heart pressures, e.g. Pulmonary artery pressure (PA pressure) using the tricuspid regurgitation velocity
- pericardial effusion – small, insignificant pericardial effusions may occur in pregnancy
- intra-cardiac shunts
- congenital heart disease.

Chamber dimensions and wall thickness (Table 3.5)

All internal dimensions are mildly increased in pregnancy, with the largest change seen in atria, see Table 3.5b. Wall thickness normally remains unchanged in pregnancy, whereas it is increased (hypertrophied) in conditions such as hypertrophic cardiomyopathy and long-standing hypertension, see Fig. 3.3. Thinner areas of the ventricular wall may be due to scarring, e.g. from a previous myocardial infarction (MI) or in dilated cardiomyopathy.

Table 3.5a Wall thickness and internal dimensions in non-pregnant women

Chamber	Non-pregnant woman (cm)
IVSd/PWd	0.6–1.2
LVIDd	3.9–5.3
RV – basal diameter	2–2.8
RV – mid-cavity diameter	2.7–3.3
RV – base-apex length	7.1–7.9
LA	2.7–3.8
RA	3–4

IVSd Interventricular septum in diastole

PWd Posterior Wall in diastole

LVIDd Left ventricular internal dimension in diastole

LVIDs Left ventricular internal dimension in systole

RV Right ventricle

LA Left atrium

RA Right atrium

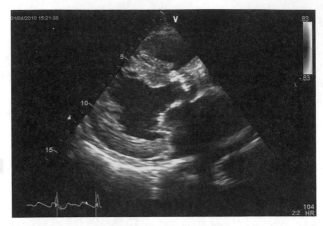

Fig. 3.3 Parasternal long axis demonstrating concentric hypertrophy.

Table 3.5b Changes in cardiac dimensions in pregnancy

	Non-pregnant	Weeks 8–12	Weeks 20–24	Weeks 30–34	Weeks 36–40
LVEDd (cm)	4	4.1	4.3	4.3	4.4
LA (cm)	2.8	3	3.2	3.3	4
RA (cm)	4.4	4.4	4.7	5.1	5.1
RVIDd (cm)	2.9	3	3.2	3.6	3.6

Left and right ventricular systolic function

The wall motion of the left and right ventricles provides a qualitative assessment of systolic function. See Table 3.6a:

Table 3.6a Descriptives used when describing ventricular wall motion

Ventricular wall motion	Example
Hyperkinetic	'Increased' contractility –physiological change often seen in pregnancy due to increased blood volume and cardiac output
Normal	All regions move in a coordinated manner and all areas contract well

Table 3.6a *Continued*

Ventricular wall motion	Example
Hypokinetic	Reduced wall motion – seen in ischaemic heart disease (IHD)/cardiomyopathy
Akinetic	Absent wall motion – seen in IHD/cardiomyopathy
Dyskinetic	Uncoordinated wall motion – commonly seen in bundle branch block

Left ventricular function

Qualitative and quantitative methods are both employed to describe left ventricular function (Table 3.6b). Quantitative assessment of left ventricular systolic function is commonly made using the ejection fraction:

$$EF = \frac{LVIDd - LVIDs}{LVIDd} \; \%$$

When interpreting LV volumes remember that blood volume increases in pregnancy and these values will be higher than non-pregnant levels.

Pregnant women with an EF < 55% should be referred to a cardiologist for assessment of possible cardiomyopathy.

Right ventricular function

Right ventricular systolic function is usually measured by observing wall motion.

Table 3.6b Echocardiographic measurements of ejection fraction and left ventricular volumes in the non-pregnant woman

	Normal	Mild impairment	Moderate impairment	Severe Impairment
LVEF	>55%	45–54%	36–44%	≤35
LV diastole volume ml	56–104	105–117	118–130	≥131
LV systole volume ml	19–49	50–59	60–69	≥70

Valves

- Mild mitral, tricuspid and pulmonary regurgitation are commonly seen in pregnancy due to the increase in mitral, tricuspid, and pulmonary annuli.
- **Beware:** a hyper-dynamic circulation and raised stroke volume increase the velocity of blood flow across valves. This results in increased systolic and diastolic gradients which may erroneously be reported as valvular disease.
- In pregnancy, a minor regurgitant leak may appear more significant due to the increased cardiac output.

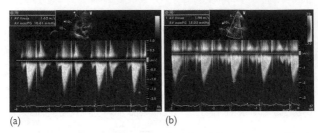

(a)   (b)

Fig. 3.4 Doppler flows across the aortic valve before a woman is pregnant (a) and when she is 12 weeks pregnant (b). Note the increase in scale in (b).

Pressure (mmHg) = 4 V^2

V= velocity across valve (m/s)

- Prosthetic valves should be carefully assessed for valve area, transvalvular gradient, paravalvular leak, and any evidence of thrombus
- Valve area, wherever possible, should be used in addition to the valve velocities and pressure gradients. This may not be possible when assessing the aortic valve area as this requires accurate measurement of the left ventricular outflow tract (LVOT).

AVA = CSA x V_1/V_2

AVA = Aortic valve area
CSA = Cross sectional area of left ventricular outflow tract cm^2
V_1 = Sub-aortic velocity m/s
V_2 = Aortic velocity m/s

- Mitral valve area may be calculated by planimetry whereby the cross-sectional area of the valve is manually traced. Again, this may not provide an accurate measurement.

Aortic valve

The normal aortic valve is composed of three leaflets. In developed countries, stenosis due to calcification from past rheumatic fever is rare. As discussed earlier, the increased velocities across the valves during pregnancy may give the false impression of stenosis. Likewise, normal physiological changes such as annulur dilatation may produce mild aortic regurgitation (AR).

Table 3.7 Echo measurements of aortic stenosis in non-pregnant women

	Normal	Mild	Moderate	Severe
Peak velocity m/s	<1.7	1.7–2.9	3–4	>4
Peak pressure gradient mmHg		<36	36–64	>64
Mean pressure gradient mmHg		<25	25–40	>40
Valve area cm^2	>2	1.5–2	1–1.4	<1

Table 3.7b Echo measurements of aortic regurgitation in non-pregnant women

	Mild	Severe
Pressure half time milliseconds	>500	>250

Mitral valve

In the developed world, where the incidence of rheumatic fever is low, mitral stenosis is uncommon in the young. However, it is still relatively common in the developing world. The changing haemodynamics in pregnancy often lead to 'decompensation' of the mitral stenosis in these women. Careful, regular monitoring of the valve function and area is required in these circumstances Table 3.8a.

Mitral regurgitation (MR) is seen to a mild extent in normal pregnancies. In conditions such as IHD or dilated cardiomyopathy it may be pathological.

Mitral valve prolapse
- Incidence is 2–3% in the healthy population.
- Usually a benign condition.
- May lead to MR in pregnancy due to mitral valve annular dilatation Table 3.8b.

Table 3.8a Echocardiographic assessment of mitral stenosis

	Normal	Mild	Moderate	Severe
Pressure half time m/s	40–70	71–139	140–219	>219
Mean pressure drop mmHg		<5	5–10	>10
Valve area cm^2	4–6	1.6–2	1.5–1	<1

Table 3.8b Grading of mitral regurgitation in the non-pregnant woman

	Mild	Moderate	Severe
Vena contracta (width of neck of regurgitant jet, cm)	<0.3		>0.7
Effective regurgitant orifice area (EROA)(cm^2)	<0.2	0.21–0.39	>0.4
Regurgitant volume (mL)	<30	31–59	≥60

Tricuspid valve

Stenosis due to rheumatic heart disease is uncommon in developed countries where tricuspid stenosis is more often associated with congenital heart disease.

Tricuspid regurgitation

A small degree of regurgitation is common in pregnancy but due to the increased cardiac output at this time, this may become more significant see Table 3.9.

As the pressure gradient of the regurgitant jet of the tricuspid valve is used when calculating pulmonary artery pressures (see below), there is the danger of falsely reporting pulmonary hypertension.

Table 3.9 Echocardiographic changes seen in tricuspid regurgitation in the non-pregnant woman.

	Mild	Moderate	Severe
Vena contracta (width of neck of regurgitant jet, cm)	Not defined	<0.7	>0.7
Continuous wave regurgitant jet density and colour	Soft/parabolic	Dense/variable	Dense/triangular
RA/RV/IVC size	Normal	Normal/dilated	Usually dilated

Echocardiography to investigate pulmonary embolism (see CTPA and V/Q scans)

British Thoracic Society guidelines recommend the use of echocardiography in the diagnosis of a massive Pulmonary Embolism (PE) when a CT pulmonary angiogram (CTPA) is not readily available or possible to perform. The characteristic echocardiographical findings of a PE are:
- raised pulmonary artery systolic pressures (PASP)
- impaired right ventricular systolic function
- dilated right ventricle.

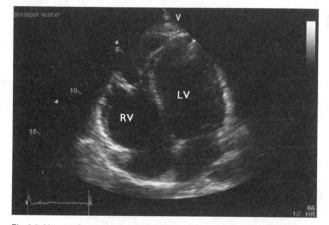

Fig. 3.5 Magnetic Resonance scan of a four chamber view with a dilated right ventricle and dilated atria.
LV = left ventricle, RV = Right ventricle, LA = left atrium, RA = right atrium.

Normal PAP is up to 25 mmHg (at rest)

Elevated PASP may cause an increase in TR. The PAP can be calculated from the tricuspid regurgitation velocity using the equation

$PAP = 4V_{tr}^2 + JVP$

V_{tr} = TR velocity

JVP= Jugular venous pressure

RAP = Right atrial pressure

The JVP is used to estimate the RAP. Likewise, the RAP can be estimated from the IVC diameter and the extent to which it collapses with inspiration. The gravid uterus presses down onto the IVC and may cause an increase in JVP height and IVC diameter. This in turn may give a misleadingly higher estimation of PAP.

The increased cardiac output seen in pregnancy may exaggerate previously mild TR, which in turn may give a high pulmonary artery pressure.

In large PEs, the PASP increases to such an extent that there is impaired systolic function and dilation of the RV.

Dobutamine stress echocardiography (DSE)

This is a non-invasive test that may be performed in those patients who cannot perform exercise. There is sparse literature regarding the use of DSE in pregnancy but no reported adverse effects, therefore it is been increasingly used.

Indications

- Determine functional capacity of patients with pre-existing cardiac disease or those with suspected coronary artery disease.
- Assess cardiac structure and function mainly in patients with aortic stenosis.

Procedure

- No caffeine or beta-blockers to be consumed 2 hours prior to the test.
- An intra-venous cannula is inserted in the hand or arm.
- A weight-adjusted dobutamine infusion is commenced and is increased until the target heart rate is reached (210-age).
- Simultaneously, a transthoracic echocardiogram is performed.
- An ECG and blood pressure is performed at different stages of the test.

Common side effects

- Chest pain
- Nausea
- Arrhythmias
- High blood pressure
- Dizzy spells

Trans-oesophageal echocardiography

This is an invasive method of imaging the heart and provides much clearer images than trans-thoracic views. It is not contra-indicated in pregnancy when the risks of missing a diagnosis, e.g. infective endocarditis outweigh the risks of the procedure.

The main problem in pregnancy is the risk of aspiration from the procedure especially in the sedated patient. Help should therefore be gained from a cardiac and/or obstetric anaesthetist who can advise on the best agents to use and be there to monitor the airway and saturations adequately. It may be necessary to perform this test under general anaesthesia.

Indications

- Assessing valvular heart disease.
- Suspected bacterial endocarditis (sensitivity with TOE = 90%, TTE = 60% in vegetations <5 mm).
- Cardiac source of emboli (endocarditis, thrombus, patent foramen ovale, myxoma).
- Congenital heart disease.

Procedure

- The patient is fasted at least 4 hours prior to the test.
- An intra-venous cannula is inserted.
- Oxygen is supplied via nasal cannulae.
- HR and oxygen saturations are monitored using a pulse oximeter.
- Lidocaine spray is used to anaesthetize the throat.
- i.v. midazolam may be required for sedation but the test can be performed without this.
- The patient lies supine in the left lateral position with the knees flexed and brought up as far as possible towards the chest.
- The transoesopheal probe is covered with a sheath, lubricated with gel and passed through the mouth, into the pharynx and then into the oesophagus and stomach where images are obtained.
- Flumazenil should be at hand to quickly reverse the effects of sedation if required.

Risks (as quoted outside pregnancy)

- 1:100 throat discomfort
- 1:1000 laryngospasm, ventricular arrhythmia, oesophageal rupture, hypoxia
- < 1:10000 deaths

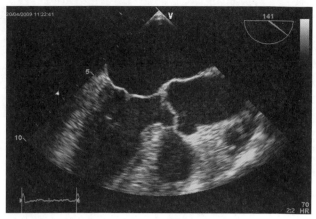

Fig. 3.6 A TOE image of the aortic and mitral valve.

Radiological investigations

There is a widely held misconception that tests involving ionizing radiation are contra-indicated in pregnant women.

The radiation dose required to either harm the fetus or cause a miscarriage is 5 Rad/50000 µGy. This far exceeds the typical dose delivered for most routine tests.

If an investigation is required for a diagnosis then there is no reason to withhold it. Clearly, one must try to limit the number of these investigations and ensure there is adequate shielding of the fetus, e.g. with a lead shield over the abdomen.

Table 3.10 Estimated radiation dose to fetus during investigations

Investigation	Dose (µGy)
CXR	<10
Limited venography with shield	<500
Perfusion lung scan technetium-99m	60–120
Ventilation lung scan technetium 99m	10–350
CT pulmonary angiography	<500
Coronary angiography (femoral)	1000*

*When performed by an experienced operator, fetal dose from a coronary angiogram procedure via the radial route is slightly lower as there is no need to screen below the diaphragm.

Chest x-ray

Common findings in normal pregnancy include:
- prominent vascular markings
- horizontal position of the heart
- flattened left heart border
- raised diaphragm due to gravid uterus
- small pleural effusions seen post-partum.

CXR findings in congestive cardiac failure
- Alveolar oedema
- Prominence of superior pulmonary veins
- Fluid in inter-lobar fissures
- Pleural effusions

Other abnormal CXR findings
- Widened mediastinum (seen in thoracic aortic dissection – note – the absence of this does not exclude a dissection). Remember however, there is slight unfolding of the aorta in normal pregnancy which may cause slight widening.
- Rib 'notching' seen in coarctation of the aorta.

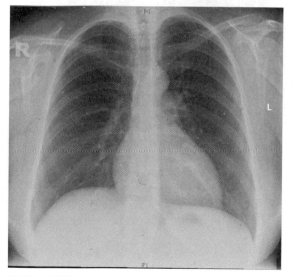

Fig. 3.7 Normal CXR of a pregnant woman.

CT pulmonary angiography (CTPA)

Commonly used as the gold-standard test to exclude a **pulmonary embolism (PE)**, this may be performed during pregnancy if required: the risk of harming the fetus due to ionizing radiation is negligible and is far out-weighed by the risk of missing a PE in the pregnant woman.

The greatest radiation exposure is to the patient (especially breast tissue) and not the fetus (see Table 3.10).

Procedure

The patient must lie supine for the test which is a problem in the latter stages of pregnancy as the pregnant uterus causes obstruction of the vena-cava.

An intra-venous cannula is used to administer 50–150ml contrast.

The CT scan takes approximately 5 minutes to acquire images.

Emboli appear as filling defects within the vasculature.

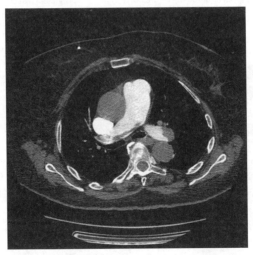

Fig. 3.8 A CT pulmonary angiogram of a pregnant woman demonstrating thrombus in the pulmonary artery.

Radionuclide investigations

These investigations involve the use of radioisotopes and may be used in pregnant women if required.

Ventilation–perfusion (V/Q) scan

This investigation, used in the diagnosis of PE, is not contra-indicated in pregnancy. The risks of radiation exposure to the fetus are negligible.

The V/Q scan detects any mismatch in the ventilation and perfusion of the lungs. A radioisotope is attached to the blood and if there is a pulmonary embolism, this appears as a perfusion defect.

Omitting the ventilation portion of the VQ scan in pregnant women, reduces the level of radiation (see Table 3.10) and is appropriate if the CXR is normal (see Figure 3.9).

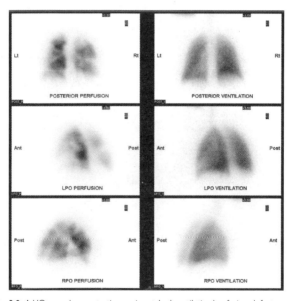

Fig. 3.9 A VQ scan demonstrating a mismatched ventilation/perfusion defects which is indicative of a pulmonary embolus.

Myocardial perfusion imaging

This is a non-invasive investigation performed to assess perfusion of the myocardium.

As there are alternatives which do not involve radio-isotopes, e.g. ETT/DSE, this has not been used in pregnancy and therefore should probably be avoided. Its analysis is subjective, and the large vascular breast may lead to excess artifact.

Cardiac magnetic resonance imaging (CMR)

The safety of CMRI in the early stages of pregnancy is not yet determined and is not routinely used in the first trimester of pregnancy but has been used in the second and third trimesters.

It has the advantage of providing detailed 3-dimensional information on cardiac anatomy and function but it is only used if other investigations such as echocardiography cannot provide the relevant information (see Figure 3.10).

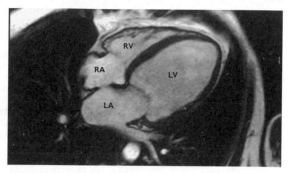

Fig. 3.10 Magnetic resonance scan showing a four chamber view with a dilated left ventricle. The left atrium is also enlarged. LV = left ventricle, RV = Right ventricle, LA = left atrium, RA = right atrium.

Invasive procedures

Implantable loop recorder

Some arrhythmias causing symptoms of palpitations, syncope or pre-syncope occur so infrequently, practically it is not possible to capture them with standard Holter recordings. In these cases, an implantable loop recorder (2 x 3 cm) can be inserted in the left pre-pectoral area using local anaesthesia.

If the patient is aware of any symptoms, then by pressing a button, they activate the device to record up to 30 minutes before and after the event.

Whilst these are not contraindicated in pregnancy, they are unlikely to be required though some women may fall pregnant having had one previously implanted. Their battery life is up to 2 years after which they can be removed at the patient's convenience.

Electrophysiological studies and radio-frequency ablation

Electrophysiological studies (EPS) are usually undertaken as part of the procedure to curatively ablate an abnormal conduction pathway (radio-frequency ablation (RFA)). They do however use a significant amount of ionising radiation thus conferring risk both to the maternal breast and fetus. In virtually all cases, the arrhythmia can be controlled with medications until after delivery. There have been case reports of women undergoing EPS and RFA for life-threatening ventricular arrhythmias. Radiation can be minimized using non-fluoroscopic catheter location systems as well as lead shielding.

Cardiac catheterization (see Chapter 4 IHD)

Indications
- Assessing and treating coronary artery disease.
- Measurements of intra-cardiac chambers and oxygen saturations.
- Performing valvular annuloplasty, e.g. for mitral stenosis.
- PFO closure.

Used with caution in pregnancy due to the high radiation exposure to the fetus, this is not contra-indicated when assessing and treating coronary artery disease. Percutanous coronary stent insertion is the gold-standard treatment for myocardial infarction due to atheroma or dissection.

Procedure
- The patient is ideally fasted for 4 hours prior to the procedure.
- Pre-procedure blood tests must be taken: FBC, U & E, clotting profile and group and save.
- The dye used is nephro-toxic and those patients with pre-existing renal disease must have adequate intra-venous hydration pre-procedure and an alternative dye (VISIPAQUE©) is used.
- The femoral or radial artery may be used for coronary artery catheterisation. In pregnant women, the gravid uterus may compress the abdominal vessels and make the procedure technically difficult via the femoral route.
- A lead shield is placed over the abdomen to reduce radiation exposure to the fetus.
- The radiation exposure to the fetus is highest when using the femoral approach significant complications.
- Risks are 1:1000 for diagnostic procedures and from 1:100 for interventional procedures outside pregnancy. These risks include myocardial infarction, bleeding/bruising, arrhythmias, stroke, renal failure, the need for urgent coronary artery bypass surgery and death.

Coronary artery catheterization
- The radial artery is the preferred route of access in pregnant women as it reduces radiation exposure to the fetus and avoids the pressure-effect of the gravid uterus.
- Under X-ray guidance, a coronary catheter is passed in to the ostium of the right and left coronary artery.
- Radio-opaque dye is injected into the artery and images are taken from different angles.
- In the case of acute coronary syndromes or myocardial infarction, the narrowed, occluded or dissected artery may be opened up by passing a wire through the occlusion.
- A balloon is inflated over the wire and then a stent is inserted.

It is increasingly successfully used in the context of primary percutaneous coronary intervention (primary PCI) to treat acute myocardial infarction. In this event, the well-being of the woman supersedes the risk of radiation exposure to the fetus.

Right heart catheterization

The right femoral vein is usually used but in pregnant patients the brachial vein may be utilized.

Both procedures may take up to 1 hour and in the advanced stages of pregnancy may not be possible as the patient must lie supine. However once the catheters have been inserted (if using the femoral route) or if using the brachial route, it is possible to tilt the pelvis laterally to move the uterus off the IVC while maintaining the chest flat against the operating table.

Conclusion

When investigating the pregnant woman with known or suspected heart disease, it is important to know the limitations of each procedure, and choose the relevant investigation after balancing diagnostic power and safety. It is crucial to understand the variance between results in and out of pregnancy, to ensure an incorrect diagnosis is not made.

Ischaemic heart disease

Epidemiology

- Ischaemic heart disease (IHD) is the commonest cause of cardiovascular death in the UK.
- Deaths from IHD are falling in non-pregnant women of childbearing age.
- Myocardial infarction (MI)/IHD is the commonest cause of cardiac mortality in pregnancy (25% of all cardiac deaths).
- Maternal deaths from MI are rising.
- Pregnancy increases the risk of MI.
- Worldwide maternal death rate from acute MI is 20%.

Pathophysiology of IHD in pregnancy

Atherosclerosis

- Affects over half of the women with MI in or around pregnancy (these women usually have risk factors—see Table 4.1).
- Affects large and medium sized vessels (from first decade of life).
- Endothelial dysfunction triggers deposition of lipid rich macrophages in the vessel walls → build up into fatty streaks → fibrous plaques.
- Stable plaques impede flow down coronary arteries → anginal symptoms.
- Unstable plaques can rupture releasing the highly thrombogenic lipid rich core → occlusive thrombus which reduces coronary perfusion → MI.

Thrombosis

- Pregnancy is a prothrombotic state and arterial thrombi can form in "at risk" individuals (see Chapter 21, Thrombo-embolic disease).
- Therefore, acute occlusion of coronary arteries due to thrombus formation can occur on otherwise angiographically normal (or endothelial intact) vessels.

Dissection

- Spontaneous coronary artery dissection is due to sheer stress along vessel walls.
- Rare outside pregnancy.
- Occurred in 3 out of the 8 deaths in 2000–2002 CEMACH report.

Risk factors

Table 4.1 Risk factors for ischaemic heart disease in pregnant women

Classic risk factors	Other risk factors in women
Family history	Increasing age
Diabetes	Ethnicity (esp SE Asian)
Hypertension	Obesity
Smoking	Physical inactivity
Hypercholesterolaemia	Multiparity

Pre-pregnancy counselling of high risk women who are not known to have coronary disease

The latest CEMACH report has stated pre-pregnancy counselling;

- Should be provided for women of child-bearing age with pre-existing serious medical condition which may be aggravated by pregnancy
- Women at higher risk of developing cardiac disease in pregnancy are defined as:
  - obese
  - smokers
  - pre-existing hypertension
  - diabetes
  - family history of FH heart disease
  - 35 years old.

These recommendations especially apply to women prior to undergoing fertility treatments.

See p. 76 for discussion on counselling a woman post coronary event.

Coronary artery disease presentations

Coronary artery disease is divided into stable 'Angina pectoris' or unstable 'Acute coronary syndromes' (ACS) (see below)

Stable coronary heart disease—angina

Symptoms

- Usually associated with exercise – pain at rest is either non-ischaemic or part of an ACS.
- A band-like pain, around the chest radiating up to the jaw or down the left arm or.
- A 'tightness' or 'ache' rather than pain.
- Never sharp.
- Not localized but distributed over an area of the chest -pin-point pain can be distinguished easily as non-cardiac.
- Lasting minutes—pain lasting seconds or longer than an hour is usually non-cardiac.
- Associated with sweatiness, nausea, fatigue, breathlessness.
- Symptoms are relieved with rest/with GTN within a minute.

Examination

- Often normal at rest when the patient has no symptoms
- Look for presence of risk factors, e.g.
  - Hypertension.
  - Xanthelasma (cholesterol deposits under the eyes).
  - Nicotine stained fingers.

Acute coronary syndromes (ACS)

Acute coronary syndrome is a term which includes the diagnosis of unstable angina (UA), non ST elevation myocardial infarction (NSTEMI) and ST elevation myocardial infarction (STEMI).

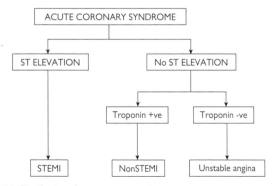

Fig. 4.1 Classification of acute coronary syndromes.

They are usually divided into two groups on the basis of their treatment:

1) ST elevation myocardial infarction STEMI (see Fig. 4.2)

- Complete occlusion of the coronary vessel.
- ST elevation on the resting ECG in association with patient's symptoms.
- Some patients suffering a STEMI do not have ST elevation in their ECG but new LBBB.
- Require immediate treatment to reperfuse the cardiac muscle.

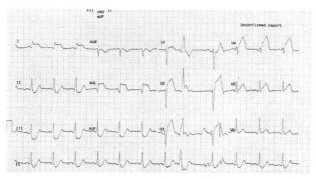

Fig. 4.2 ECG of anterior STEMI. Note clear ST elevation V_2 to V_5 with reciprocal ST depression II, III and avf, anterior.

2) Non ST elevation myocardial infarction NSTEMI (see Fig. 4.3)
- Incomplete occlusion of the coronary vessel.
- Plaque ruptures causing severely reduced flow leading to ischaemia of the cardiac muscle, but the vessel is still open.
- Symptoms may come and go, depending upon the formation and resolution of platelet aggregation and thrombus formation.
- Typical ECG changes are ST depression or dynamic T wave inversion.
- If there is biochemical evidence of myocardial damage (usually raised troponin – see p. 65) then the term used is NSTEMI whereas if the cardiac enzymes are normal the term used is unstable angina.

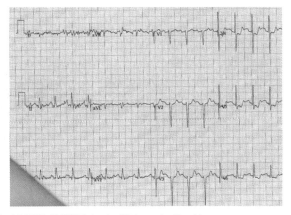

Fig. 4.3 ECG of NSTEMI showing ST depression V_4 to V_6.

Presentation of ACS
- Often no prior history of cardiac symptoms.
- Acute onset of symptoms – chest pain often more intense and severe than angina, occurs on minimal exertion or at rest, and patients usually feel very unwell.
- Chest pain often associated with other symptoms, e.g. nausea and vomiting, breathlessness, feeling clammy and sweaty and may include pre-syncope or syncope.
- ACS chest pain may initially be ignored by the patient, presuming it to be a severe bout of indigestion, and this may be a problem in the pregnant woman.
- If a pregnant woman calls a midwife or labour ward for advice about chest pain or indigestion, they should be advised to attend hospital for assessment.

Diagnosis of coronary artery disease
The diagnosis of ACS is made on the basis of a history of:
- Chest pain, with
  - ECG changes
  - Positive cardiac markers: troponins (see Chapter 3 p. 29).

CK/CKMB is less reliable than troponins.

Troponin levels are higher in women with pre-eclampsia compared to normotensive pregnant women; however, they **DO NOT** reach the threshold for diagnosis of an ACS outside pregnancy.

Troponin levels peak after 12 hours post event though may be detectable as early as 6 hours. To prevent the need to re-test and to avoid false negative results, troponin levels are thus taken 12 or greater hours post event. They remain elevated for up to 14 days post event.

Stable angina is diagnosed using:
- history compatible with angina +/−
- evidence of ischaemia on non-invasive testing OR
- positive coronary angiogram (unlikely to be done in pregnant woman before non-invasive testing).

Investigations

The normal investigations are discussed further in Chapter 3.

ECG

Resting ECG often normal unless previous event where may be any of the following abnormalities: (see Figure 3.2)
- T wave inversion in contiguous leads
- LBBB
- residual ST elevation
- pathological 'Q' waves.

Blood test results

- Troponins are normal in pregnancy (see above and Chapter 3 p. 29).
- Other blood tests may be abnormal revealing cause of chest pain e.g. HELLP syndrome (see p. 199 Hypertension).
- It is not useful to measure cholesterol in pregnancy as it is raised by 40–60% in normal pregnancy.

Non-invasive assessment of coronary arteries

- Provides objective evidence if cardiac chest pain is suspected.
- In pregnancy, the tests most commonly used are those which avoid radiation:
  - exercise treadmill testing (ETT) – Readily available and simple to do but high false positive rate in women (see p. 32)
  - dobutamine stress echo (DSE) – Less readily available but greater accuracy in high volume operators if good images can be obtained (see p. 43).
- Myocardial perfusion scanning involves a nuclear medicine technique and therefore should be avoided in pregnant women.
- CT coronary angiography is not really used in pregnant women, because if she is to be exposed to radiation, then standard coronary angiography should be performed as it also allows for intervention at the same time, thus minimizing overall radiation.

Invasive assessment of coronary arteries—coronary angiography

- Perform if coronary artery disease is suspected in pregnancy.
- Concern about fetal and maternal breast radiation is outweighed by fatality risk of undiagnosed and potentially untreated coronary disease.
- Minimize maternal and fetal radiation risk by using the radial rather than the femoral artery, fetal shielding, limited views and radiation, low ionic contrast.
- Coronary angiography can be immediately followed by treatment if required i.e. coronary artery angioplasty.

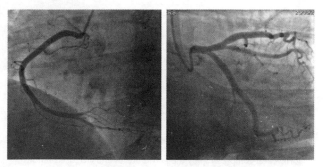

Fig. 4.4a and b Fig. 4.4a is a normal right coronary artery (RCA) and Fig. 4.4b is a normal left coronary artery (LCA).

Initial management of ACS

- All women with suspected ACS should be monitored in an area with fully trained staff and full resuscitation facilities available, particularly defibrillators. This is usually best done either in a resuscitation area of an emergency department or coronary care.
- Continuous cardiac monitoring is essential.
- Give 300 mg aspirin stat, if not already administered by the paramedics.

Immediate management should involve:

- high flow oxygen
- venous access (at least 18G cannula)
- nurse woman in the left lateral position if over 20 weeks to relieve aorto-caval compression by the gravid uterus and increased venous return
- pain relief—usually diamorphine 2.5–5 mg IV given with anti-emetic e.g. cyclizine 50 mg IV
- 12 lead ECG to confirm diagnosis and allow treatment decision
- rapid examination to exclude hypotension, note murmurs, diagnose and treat pulmonary oedema
- The administration of clopidogrel 600 mg (if the woman is currently pain free with no significant ECG changes then a loading dose of 300 mg can be used instead). This is given in addition to aspirin.

Treatment of STEMI

- The mainstay of treatment in STEMI patients is rapid reperfusion of the infarct territory which is marked by resolution of the ST elevation. Currently there are two main ways this is achieved in the UK: thrombolytic therapy or primary percutaneous coronary angioplasty (PPCI). The procedure is described further in this chapter on page 71
- It is beyond the scope of this book to debate the pros and cons of each outside pregnancy but in summary, PPCI has been proven to be superior to thrombolytic therapy provided it can be offered in a timely fashion which necessitates 24hour access to cardiac catheter laboratory facilities.

PPCI

In pregnancy there are two main reasons why PPCI should be favoured over thrombolysis if it can be delivered, ideally within 90 minutes of presentation:

- thrombolysis is associated with a significant risk of bleeding and this can cause catastrophic haemorrhage in the woman with resultant fetal loss
- outside pregnancy, bleeding is seen in 10% of patients usually at puncture sites with major bleeds seen in up to 1% of patients
- STEMI associated with pregnancy may be due to coronary dissection which is best treated by PCI and may be aggravated by thrombolysis.

Unfractionated heparin (70 units per kg) is given peri-procedure. There is still a risk of bleeding associated with the procedure but less than that associated with thrombolytic therapy.

Thrombolysis

- Use if PPCI is not available—ideally given within 30 mins of presentation.
- If a women presents late (after 6 hours of onset of symptoms) she is best discussed with a cardiologist as the benefits from thrombolysis are reduced.
- The choice of thrombolytic should be governed by normal local policy as there are no data in pregnancy comparing the different agents.
  - Streptokinase is associated with a higher risk of allergic reactions (particularly after repeat administration) and hypotension.
  - Recombinant tissue plasminogen activator (rtPA) has marginally higher survival outside pregnancy BUT an increased risk of haemorrhage.

Treatment of NSTEMI

Patients with NSTEMI who do not require immediate transfer to the cardiac catheter lab should also receive:

- low molecular weight heparin (LMWH)
  - this has been shown to be superior to unfractionated heparin (UFH) in the management of ACS and is easier to administer.
  - it is used extensively in pregnancy in the prevention and treatment of thromboembolic disease and does not cross the placenta so is safe for the fetus. (see anticoagulation Chapter 17).
  - continue LMWH for at least 2 days after the last episode of chest pain or dynamic ECG changes.
  - if there is concern over bleeding, UFH can be used, however, it is difficult to accurately titrate and higher doses than in the non-pregnant woman are required to obtain an APTT ratio between 2 and 2.5.
- GIIbIIIa receptor inhibitor
  - This further anti-platelet drug is given to patients with high risk lesions, e.g. poor flow, dissections, high thrombus load.
  - Abiciximab or tirofihan are most commonly used in the UK. However, tirofiban and eptifibatide have received FDA category B recommendation, whereas ReoPro is a category C (see Table 19.1, p.255).
  - this comes as an IV infusion and is given on a weight adjusted basis. Whilst each case has to be assessed on its individual merits, the authors we recommend trying to avoid its use in the pregnant woman as the effects on the fetus are unknown, plus the benefit gained will probably be outweighed by the significant extra bleeding risk.
  - if considered essential for the safe outcome of mother, tirofiban or eptifibatide have the greatest safety data in pregnancy.

Further anti-ischaemic therapy for IHD patients includes:
- beta-blockers – Metoprolol has the most safety data but high doses are often required in pregnancy to achieve HR reduction. Bisoprolol (2.5–10 mg) atenolol is a good alternative (25–50 mg od).
- calcium channel blockers – use verapamil or amlodipine.
- nitrates.

Percutaneous coronary intervention (PCI)

If significant coronary lesions are identified that require intervention then the women would go onto have a PCI (also known as coronary angioplasty). This involves passing a fine wire down the coronary artery, dilating the lesion with a balloon and securing the lesion with a stent (a metal scaffold) see Fig. 4.5.

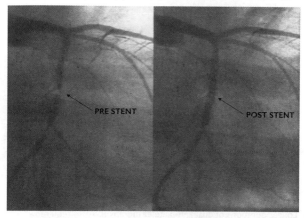

Fig. 4.5 A significant stenosis (left panel) is stented with good result (right panel).

Coronary stents

Stents broadly come in two forms, bare metal stents (BMS) or drug eluting stents (DES)—see Table 4.2.

Bare metal stents (BMS)

Advantages

- Stent endothelialized within 1 month of insertion → no 'bare metal' is exposed to passing blood and platelets → reduced risk of thrombosis.
- Only one month of a second antiplatelet agent (clopidogrel) required in addition to low dose (75 mg) aspirin: useful in pregnancy where bleeding at delivery and post-partum is a concern.

Disadvantages

- Increased in stent-restenosis (ISR):
  - smooth muscle proliferation as a 'healing mechanism' within the artery → reduction in lumen size and hence reduction in coronary blood flow
  - usually presents around 3–6 months after stent insertion.

Drug eluting stents (DES)

These are metal stents with an active drug attached to them via a polymer which elutes into the artery after deployment to reduce in-stent restenosis.

Advantages

- Reduced ISR.

Disadvantages

- Increased thrombotic risk.
- Longer durations of dual anti-platelet therapy (DAPT) required - clopidogrel for 12 months after stent deployment.
- Resultant significant bleeding risks particularly at delivery and post-partum due to DAPT.
- **Premature discontinuation of clopidogrel is associated with an increased risk of stent thrombosis which can lead to MI and death**.

Irrespective of type of stent used, patients whom have had an ACS have improved mortality and morbidity when treated with 12 months clopidogrel.

As there are no data available to guide the cardiologist as to the pros and cons of each stent, decisions need to be taken on an individual basis.

Table 4.2 Comparison between bare metal stents and drug eluting stents

	Bare metal stent	Drug eluting stent
Stent endothelialization	One month	Longer
Stent thrombosis risk	+	++
Aspirin 75 mg	✓	✓
Clopidogrel duration	One month	One year
In stent re-stenosis rate	++	+

Coronary artery bypass grafting (CABG)

Whilst this is widely used for the treatment of coronary artery disease, it is often not required in the younger patient. Cardiac surgery carries significant risk of maternal and fetal mortality (see Chapter 8).

Implications for delivery

Mode of delivery

- As highlighted many times in this book, and discussed in detail in Chapter 24, p. 310, vaginal delivery offers a safer mode of delivery for the majority of patients, including women with IHD and ACS.
- Beta-blockers should be continued throughout labour to prevent a significant increase in heart rate and BP.
- If there are concerns about the woman, the second stage should be assisted with a ventouse or forceps.

Analgesia in labour

- Whilst epidural is the preferred method of analgesia by many women, the majority of anaesthetists will be reluctant to site an epidural in a woman on dual antiplatelet therapy because of the risk of bleeding and epidural haematoma. This is another reason for wishing to discontinue clopidogrel prior to delivery.
- Women should be counselled about this and given the chance to discuss alternative methods with their midwife and obstetric anaesthetist.

Uterotonics

- The risk of post-partum haemorrhage is increased in women on aspirin and clopidogrel. The third stage of labour should be actively managed and in those on clopidogrel or dual antiplatelet therapy, a prophylactic infusion of syntocinon should be administered.
  - Syntocinon can be used to augment labour if necessary. For an active third stage, 5 iu should be mixed in 20 ml of normal saline and administered slowly (over 20 minutes). For post-partum haemorrhage treatment or prevention, it can be administered as an infusion, as with non-cardiac women.
  - Ergometrine and syntometrine® should be avoided (cause hypertension).
  - Misoprostol 800–1000 mcg rectally can be used for post-partum haemorrhage.
  - Carboprost 250 mcg can be used for post-partum haemorrhage.
  - Surgical methods may be required (see Chapter 24).

Risk and counselling in future pregnancy

- Patients who are post ACS are usually discharged on aspirin, clopidogrel (for 12 months), an ACE inhibitor, beta-blocker, and a statin. Whilst aspirin and beta-blockers can be used in pregnancy, ACE inhibitors and statins are contraindicated. Women should be counselled that these will need to be discontinued prior to a future pregnancy.
- Premature cessation of anti-platelet therapy, which may be necessary around delivery, is associated with risk of stent thrombosis. Ideally pregnancy should be delayed to avoid this risk.
- Women with known IHD should be assessed prior to conceiving to confirm they have no on-going ischaemia or significant residual disease, which should be addressed prior to pregnancy, to reduce the risk of a further ACS.
- Whilst there are no guidelines to advise how long after an ACS or coronary intervention a woman may undergo a pregnancy, the authors recommend a year to allow full recovery and cardiac remodelling, as well as assessment prior to pregnancy. When in-stent restenosis occurs, it is within the first 6 months following stent implantation.
- The overall risk is dependent upon the presence of residual ischaemia/ significant disease as well as overall LV function.
- It is important to counsel women of childbearing age who have had an event of the above risks and ensure they have adequate and appropriate contraception.

Native valvular heart disease

Native valvular heart disease affecting women of child bearing age can be either congenital or acquired. The most common cause of acquired valvular heart disease is rheumatic heart disease.

Rheumatic heart disease

Acute rheumatic fever is rare in the UK and is usually contracted in childhood.

In developing countries it is reducing but still accounts for almost half of the cardiac disease in the developing world.

Pathology and clinical features

- It typically occurs 3 to 4 weeks following a streptococcal pharyngitis.
- The most common organism is a group A beta haemolytic streptococcus, e.g. *streptococcus pyogenes*.

Patients complain of:
- fever
- abdominal pain
- migratory polyarthritis.

and depending upon the severity:
- complications of chorea
- skin rashes (erythema marginatum)
- subcutaneous nodules can occur in varying degrees.

When the heart is affected it is usually in the form of a pan-carditis.
- Pericarditis causes pain but usually no haemodynamic instability
- Myocarditis may cause acute heart failure and arrhythmias.

Endocarditis affects the mitral valve most commonly followed by the aortic valve alone, both in combination and occasionally the tricuspid valve. The pulmonary valve is rarely affected.

Valvular heart disease secondary to rheumatic heart disease therefore presents as:
- acute regurgitation and heart failure or
- chronically as either valvular regurgitation or stenosis.

Rheumatic heart disease may present for the first time in pregnancy, particularly in immigrant women who may never have previously undergone cardiovascular examination.

In the UK, mitral stenosis accounts for 90% of rheumatic heart disease in pregnancy.

Treatment

Treatment is with:
- penicillin (Erythromycin in the penicillin allergic patient)
- high dose aspirin added until inflammatory markers normalise
- moderate to severe carditis may be improved with steroid therapy whilst standard heart failure treatments are given for those in acute failure.

Congenital valvular heart disease

Aortic valve

- Bicuspid aortic valve is the most common congenital cardiac anomaly.
- It affects 1–2% of the population with a 4:1 male:female preponderance
- 20% of patients have other anomalies, e.g. aortic coarctation, PDA
- Severity tends to increase with age with chance of aortic valve replacement (AVR) being 1% in first decade of life to 30% in 7th decade (age 60–69).

Mitral valve

- Congenital mitral valve abnormalities are rare.

Pulmonary valve

- Congenital pulmonary valve abnormalities can occur in isolation but usually part of a syndrome, e.g. Noonan syndrome.
- Mild PS (<30 mmHg) rarely progresses and approx 20% moderate lesions progress to require intervention.

Tricuspid valve

- Congenital TR is associated with Ebstein's anomaly which is rare.
- Tricuspid atresia results in a complex case of a functionally univentricular heart.

General principles in pregnancy

- Regurgitant lesions are usually well tolerated and fall into the low risk category providing left ventricular function is good.
- Stenotic lesions may pose a greater problem.
  - Mild stenosis can be well tolerated.
  - Severe left sided obstruction at either the aortic valve or mitral valve is a high risk case where mortality can be higher than 10%.
  - These women are therefore advised to have their lesion corrected before embarking on a pregnancy.

As with many conditions, patients are best assessed prior to pregnancy, but if that is not possible, they should be reviewed as early as possible by a cardiologist with an interest in obstetric cardiology. This allows full understanding of the risks involved with the pregnancy to both mother and fetus as well as planning appropriate management both antenatally and during delivery.

Risk of endocarditis

This is discussed further in Chapter 6 but essentially, antibiotic prophylaxis is no longer recommended to cover delivery.

Aortic stenosis (AS)

Cause
- Most frequently as a result of congenital bicuspid valve.
- May also occur in rheumatic heart disease.
  - The aortic valve is the second most common valve to be affected in rheumatic heart disease.

REMEMBER: Bicuspid aortic valve is associated with coarctation so this must be excluded.

Presentation
Mild: This is usually asymptomatic and picked up as a result of the increased volume of the murmur due to the increased flow dynamics of pregnancy.

Moderate: Patients may experience:
1. reduction in exercise tolerance
2. shortness of breath.

Severe: Patients become increasingly symptomatic particularly in pregnancy as the fixed obstruction does not allow the physiological changes to occur as normal. Symptoms that are particularly worrying are:
- chest pain
- syncope or pre-syncope.

Physical signs
- Slow rising, low volume pulse.
- Narrow pulse pressure (small difference between systolic and diastolic BP).
- Heaving apex beat.
- May have a systolic thrill.
- Critical AS is characterized on auscultation by the lack of a second HS (A2) though in younger women, this may be confusing as the valve is more pliable therefore an ejection click may be heard. Second heart sound normal in mild AS (after sound of closure of pulmonary valve—P2) and coincides with P2 in moderate AS.
- Ejection systolic murmur, often heard throughout the praecordium and radiates to carotids. As severity worsens, the murmur lengthens and hence obscures the second heart sound.

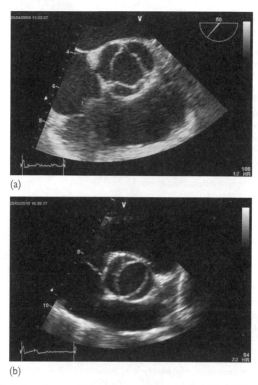

(a)

(b)

Fig. 5.1 a) shows the normal tricuspid valve whereas the valve below (b) is bicuspid.

Investigation

ECG—LVH and left axis deviation in severe AS (see Figure 5.2)

Echocardiogram—This will allow:

1. confirmation of valve morphology (bicuspid or tricuspid)
2. severity of gradient across valve
3. presence or absence of associated aortic root dilatation
4. presence or absence of associated features, e.g. coarctation, PDA
5. Confirmation of LV function – impaired LV function is a concern.

ETT (see Chapter 2):

Pre-pregnancy

- Some cardiologists advocate exercise testing in moderate-to-severe asymptomatic AS to help decide on need for intervention.
- This should always be medically supervised by cardiologists familiar with management of such cases.
- Bad prognostic signs are either:
  - ST segment change
  - failure to mount an appropriate BP rise.
- Intervention is indicated with the above features.
- May be useful in women presenting in early pregnancy to predict how the women will cope with the physiological changes of pregnancy.

MRI should be performed in cases of aortic root dilatation or where coarctation is known or suspected.

Management

General principles

- Severe lesions should be corrected prior to conception.
- Women respond well to bedrest and therefore often require admission.
- Close monitoring is required if they have a severe lesion or are symptomatic.
- Hypertension should be managed as discussed in Chapter 15.
- Beta-blockers can be very helpful with these women and are essential in those with dilated aortic roots.
  - By reducing heart rate, they increase the time the valve is open to allow greater flow through it as well as prolonging diastole and allowing greater coronary perfusion.
- Avoid drugs which reduce after load, e.g. nitrates,

Intervention is usually AVR. Balloon valvuloplasty is rarely indicated in adults but may allow safe delivery of the fetus in women running into trouble.

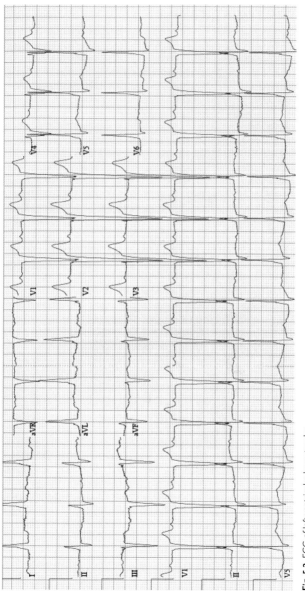

Fig. 5.2 ECG of left ventricular hypertrophy.

Aortic regurgitation

Cause
- Some bicuspid aortic valves may present with regurgitation but often in association with stenosis.
- Dilated aortic root (most common cause in young women = Marfan syndrome).
- Infective endocarditis.
- Acute aortic dissection.

Presentation
- Breathlessness.
- Symptoms of heart failure.
- Chest pain due to lack of flow down coronary arteries.

Examination
- Pulse collapsing (felt at the radial).
- Wide pulse pressure (large difference between systolic and diastolic BP).
- Apex becomes displaced with severe AR—hyperdynamic.
- May feel thrill.
- Classical signs of severe AR may be present:
  - Corrigans sign (Visible carotid pulsation)
  - Quinkes sign (visible capillary pulsation in nail bed)
  - De Musset's sign (head nodding with each pulse)
  - pistol shot femorals (loud noise heard over femoral artery when auscultated with stethoscope).
- AR murmur is a high pitched early diastolic murmur heard best at the left sternal edge at end expiration with the woman leant forward.
  - The more severe the AR the greater the length of the murmur.
- An Austin flint murmur (low pitched rumbling mid-diastolic murmur) may also be heard at the apex due to the regurgitant jet hitting the mitral valve.

Investigations
- ECG: Left axis deviation.
- CXR: In severe chronic AR the heart can become dilated leading to an increased cardiac silhouette. Aortic dilatation may also be seen.
- Echo: 2D can look at the valve function, measurements of LV and aorta can be taken and the colour and continuous wave Doppler allows for quantification of severity.

Management
Mild/moderate: usually well tolerated—may need diuretics if patient becomes SOB.

Severe: Monitor for signs of heart failure and treat with diuretics and vasodilators as required.

Mitral stenosis

- Not uncommon to present for the first time in pregnancy due to the relative tachycardia and haemodynamic changes of pregnacy.
- Rheumatic heart disease has re-emerged as a cause of maternal mortality in the UK.
- The signs may be difficult to elicit in the sick woman, and if not considered at diagnosis can be missed.

Cause

- Rheumatic fever is the main cause.
- All others are rare.

Haemodynamics

To understand the presentation of patients and problems in pregnancy, it is important to understand the haemodynamics of the lesion (see Fig. 5.4):
- stenosis of the valve leads to elevated left atrial pressure, which in turn leads to an increase in pulmonary artery pressure
- this can lead to right heart strain and failure
- the left ventricle meanwhile does not have adequate filling, which leads to a fall in cardiac output
- all these changes are made worse by the onset of tachycardia or AF as not only is there a loss of atrial systole, but decreased time for the ventricle to fill due to the increase in HR associated with the arrhythmia.

Rapid deterioration with pulmonary oedema can be prevented and reversed in these women with the use of beta-blockers (see Fig. 5.4).

Presentation

- SOB on exertion, PND, or orthopnea.
- Acute pulmonary oedema.
- Palpitations.
- Fatigue.
- Systemic embolism from AF/dilated LA.
- Chest pain.
- Symptoms from compression of a structure by enlarged LA
  - Hoarse voice (laryngeal nerve).
  - Dysphagia (oesophagus).

Physical signs

- General: Malar flush (less obvious to see in the pregnant women due to the relative vasodilation).
- Pulse: Small volume if SR, may be in AF.
- JVP: Prominent 'a' waves.
- Apex: Tapping, non-displaced.
- Left parasternal heave.
- Auscultation: loud S1 (providing patient in SR and valve pliable).
  - Opening snap.
  - Low pitch mid-diastolic murmur.

- Best heard with woman in left lateral position.
- Early diastolic murmur may be heard if patient has raised pulmonary pressures.

Investigations
- ECG—AF common but if SR, may have large bifid p waves.
- CXR—Straight left heart border, signs of pulmonary hypertension, i.e. large pulmonary arteries, evidence of pulmonary oedema.
- TTE—Valve leaflets can be seen on 2D fixed at commisures causing valve to dome. Doppler trace across valve can estimate valve area and transvalvular gradient (see Chapter 3 p. 37). Essential to assess suitability of valve for balloon valvuloplasty and thus the degree of MR if any.
- TOE—May not be required in pregnancy but does give better anatomical information, as well as assessing thrombus in LA (particularly LA appendage) if patient in AF.
- Cardiac catheterization—This allows measurement of pressures in the heart. Unlikely to be used in pregnancy unless undergoing percutaneous balloon mitral valvuloplasty (PBMV) when it would be integrated into the procedure (see Figure 5.3).

Poor prognostic features in a woman with MS are:
- severe MS as assessed by valve area <1 cm^2
- presence of moderate to severe symptoms prior to starting pregnancy.

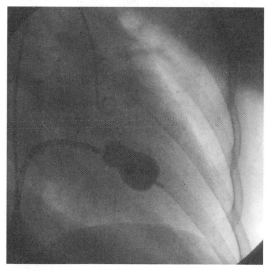

Fig. 5.3 Percutaneous balloon mitral valvuloplasty.

Treatment
- Based upon presence of symptoms, degree of stenosis and presence of any complications.
- Drugs:
  - diuretics to off load patient if has any symptoms, e.g. SOB, fatigue
  - beta-blockers to control rate, vital especially if patient in AF (see Figure 5.4)
  - digoxin can be used in woman who cannot tolerate beta-blockers but it is not as effective
  - if patient has enlarged LA, consider prophylactic LMWH
  - therapeutic LMWH should be given if the woman in AF
- Percutaneous balloon mitral valvaloplasty (PBMV)
  - this should be considered in women who are symptomatic with severe MS and a favourable valve, i.e. no significant MR, a pliable valve that is not heavily calcified, etc.
  - should be done in tertiary centre by operator with expertise in this procedure
- surgery is not often required but for further information (see Chapter 8).

Implications for delivery
- If patient is symptomatic or has severe MS, deliver in high risk centre.
- Judicious use of fluids.
- Avoid the supine and lithotomy positions.
- Try and maintain HR using beta-blockers, IV if necessary.
- Limit second stage with assisted delivery.
- Treat pulmonary oedema with oxygen, diamorphine, and diuretics.

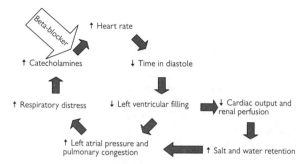

Fig. 5.4 Beta-blockers in mitral stenosis.
Reproduced with permission from Lefroy and Adamson (2007) Heart rhythm disorders. In: Oakley and Warnes, eds. *Heart Disease in Pregnancy*. Wiley–Blackwell.

Mitral regurgitation

Cause
- Infective endocarditis.
- Mitral valve prolapse.
- Rheumatic fever.
- Functional secondary to left ventricular dilation.

Presentation
- Fatigue.
- Exertional SOB.
- Palpitations (greater risk of AF).
- Pulmonary oedema.

Examination
- Tachycardia may be present.
- Displaced apex—may be forceful.
- Thrill if severe.
- Soft 1st heart sound.
- Pan-systolic murmur radiating to apex.

Investigation
- ECG—AF common in chronic MR but not seen frequently in the young.
- CXR—Cardiomegaly, LA enlargement, pulmonary congestion/oedema.
- TTE—Dilated LA, hyperdynamic LV which enlarges in severe MR Colour flow can detect severity of MR (if severe pulmonary vein flow reversal seen).
- TOE—Often used to delineate anatomy further when considering surgery so usually avoided in pregnancy.
- Cardiac catheterization—Not required in pregnancy unless considering surgery.

Management
- As with all regurgitant lesions, MR is usually well tolerated in pregnant women.
- Diuretics can be used for those with pulmonary congestion.
- Hydralazine and nitrates also can be used to off-load the ventricle.

Infective endocarditis

Introduction

- Infective endocarditis (IE) is rare in pregnancy. However, when it occurs it can be fatal for both mother and fetus.
- Whilst IE is usually associated with valvular heart disease, intra-cardiac infections can also occur on septal defects, shunts and baffles, AV malformations, and the endocardium. Infection can also occur on normal heart valves (particularly tricuspid) in women who are IV drug abusers.
- Women are thought to be at greater risk of endocarditis in pregnancy for two main reasons:
  - pregnancy is an immunocompromised state
  - certain infections, e.g. UTIs are more common in pregnancy.
- Despite this, the incidence of IE in pregnancy appears to be low with estimates around 0.03–0.14 per 1000 deliveries. Mortality, however, is high with approx 1:5 mothers dying.
- In the non-pregnant population, the greatest cause of IE is *staphylococcus aureus* whilst in the pregnant population, *streptococcus* is 3 times more common that *staphylococcus*.

Diagnostic criteria

- High index of suspicion is required in pregnancy.
- Diagnostic criteria are the same as in the non-pregnant state (see Box 6.1 and Figure 6.1).

Predisposing factors

- The incidence of bacteraemia in pregnancy is not known.
- The risk with a vaginal delivery is 0–5% and with a caesarean section is up to 14%.
- Women having a caesarean section who have not laboured have a lower risk.
- Urethral catheterization appears to be the highest risk at 18–33%.
- Women with a history of IVDU or who have had previous IE are at high risk of IE. Prosthetic heart valves, complex congenital HD with and without surgical conduits pose the highest risk.

Box 6.1

MAJOR CRITERIA

- Positive blood cultures - >2 +ve cultures with a typical organism, e.g. *strep viridans* or *staph aureus* in the absence of a primary focus (e.g. pneumonia).
- Echocardiographic features of endocardial involvement.
  - Vegetation on valve.
  - Abscess.
  - New dehiscence of prosthetic material.
  - New valve regurgitation.

MINOR CRITERIA

- Predisposing cardiac condition or intravenous drug use (IVDU) history.
- Fever > 38 °C.
- Vascular features e.g. emboli or mycotic aneurysms.
- Immunological features, e.g. glomerulonephritis and Oslers nodes.
- Positive blood cultures but not meeting major criteria.

Definite endocarditis =   2 major criteria
                                OR 1 major and 3 minor criteria
                                OR 5 minor criteria
OR pathology / bacteriological evidence from a vegetation or emboli

Possible endocarditis =   1 major and 1 minor criteria
                                OR 3 minor criteria

Adapted from Li JS, Sexton DJ, Mick N, et al. (2000) Proposed modifications to the Duke criteria for the diagnosis of infective endocarditis. *Clin Infect Dis* **30**, 633–8 and Durack DT. (1998) Approach to diagnosis of infective endocarditis. *Clin Microbiol Infect* **4** Suppl 3, 53–59.

Antibiotic prophylaxis

- Recent NICE guidelines have recommended that women undergoing obstetric procedures no longer require antibiotics to prevent IE.
- These procedures include:
  - urinary catheterization
  - amniocentesis
  - chorionic villus sampling
  - normal vaginal delivery
  - assisted vaginal delivery (ventouse or forceps)
  - caesarean section.
- Women with prolonged rupture of membranes and those having a caesarean section will receive antibiotics to prevent chorioamnionitis, endometritis and wound infection.

Management

- If IE is suspected then it is essential to obtain blood cultures (BC) preferably prior to antibiotic administration.
- There should be at least 3 sets taken, preferably 6 and they should be separated in venesection location and time (i.e. don't take them all from one vein and then put into separate bottles).
- It is paramount that a rigorous sterile technique is used to prevent contamination.
- Once BC are obtained, antibiotics can be given on advice from the local microbiology unit and are usually broad spectrum until an organism is identified and its sensitivity to antibiotics established.
- Cardiology opinion should be sought early and echocardiography is required to assess valve lesions. Remember, IE is not an echo diagnosis and a negative study does not exclude the diagnosis.

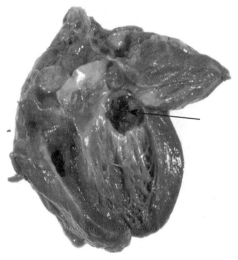

Fig. 6.1 Single image of infected mitral valve. Courtesy of Dr Andrew Deaner.

Pregnancy post cardiac surgery

Introduction

- Managing the pregnant woman who has undergone previous cardiac surgery requires a multidisciplinary approach and it is important that joint antenatal care is carried out with a high-risk obstetric team.
- Pregnancy presents a specific set of problems particularly in the context of anticoagulation and there is often a conflict of interest between the interests of the mother and the fetus and as such management may be difficult.

Cardiac surgical patients you may expect to look after are:
- post valve surgery patients
  - prosthetic valves
  - valve repair
  - surgical valvotomy
- post cardiac transplantation (see p. 150)
- post congenital surgery (see Chapters 13 and 14).

Prosthetic heart valves

There are two categories of replacement valves used in current practice:
- bioprosthetic
- metallic.

There are pros and cons for each in young women.

Bioprosthetic

These valves are 'tissue' valves and originate either from animal pericardium (bovine or porcine) or human explants, e.g. homografts.

Advantage: No need for anticoagulation.

Disadvantage: Limited durability compared to mechanical valves and thus a second operation may be necessary (approximately 80% at 10 years).

Re-do cardiac surgery carries an increased morbidity and mortality and this needs to be taken into account when considering which valve would be best suited to the individual.

Metallic

- Metallic valves are highly durable valves lasting a lifetime.
- In the western world, virtually all metallic valves implanted are bileaflet valves.
- They require life-long anticoagulation with an INR 3.5 to 4.5 times the normal range.

Problems in pregnancy

- Warfarin is teratogenic.
- The need for high levels of anticoagulation in the pregnant woman.
- An increased risk of valve thrombosis with disastrous and potentially fatal consequences.
- Warfarin crosses the placenta and therefore the fetus is anticoagulated.
- Increased risk of miscarriage fetal intra-cranial haemorrhage and stillbirth.

Valve repair

- This procedure may be preferred by surgeons to formal valve replacement in order to allow a young woman to have a family before usually requiring a further more definitive procedure.
- A repair should be successful in over 95% of women with a non-rheumatic aetiology and between 50 and 80% in a rheumatic valve.
- The main concern post surgery in these women is that the valve can often deteriorate and regurgitation is usually the prevailing problem though occasionally they stenose (particularly if they develop endocarditis). Freedom from re-operation within the child bearing period is approximately 90% but this is very variable depending upon the individual circumstances. These women should be clinically assessed in the same way as a native valve as described in Chapter 5.

Surgical mitral valvotomy

Percutaneous balloon mitral valvuloplasty (PBMV) has superseded open valvotomy of the mitral valve on the whole, though women, particularly from Indian sub-continent are still presenting having had open valvotomies. The main problem is that the valve restenoses and therefore women may re-present with functional MS. As with PBMV, mitral regurgitation can be a by product of the surgery and this may also progress over time.

Surgical aortic valvotomy

This procedure is for severe AS in a congenitally abnormal valve, i.e. bicuspid valve. However, it is very rarely carried out now as most patients can have valvuloplasty. The main problem is the re-development of aortic stenosis or aortic regurgitation.

Valve assessment

History

- It is very important to take a history and understand a woman's pre-pregnancy baseline functional state.
- Most of the symptoms of worsening valve disease can be found in the normal pregnant woman, e.g. fatigue, breathlessness, chest pain (in the normal pregnant women secondary to indigestion).

Examination

- The physical signs of a valve are similar to that of the lesion in a native valve and thus will not be discussed here individually, i.e. paravalvular leak of an aortic valve causing AR will have the signs of AR as discussed on p. 86 (see Chapter 5).
- If the woman is well, physical examination may be normal though there is often a flow murmur across a prosthetic valve.
- In prosthetic valves, the timing of the murmur is dependent upon when the valve is open, e.g. the murmur will be in systole for the aortic and pulmonary valve and diastole for the mitral and tricuspid valve. This is most pronounced with the Starr Edwards valve as the ball travels up and down the cage.
  - Other murmurs may therefore represent valvular or para-valvular (around the valve) leak, or an increasingly stenosed valve.
- Bioprosthetic valves may have normal heart sounds though this becomes more abnormal as the valve becomes less pliable.
- A metallic valve will have a higher pitched metallic sound during closure and occasionally it can be heard at opening. Valve thrombosis often fixes the valve in an open or closed position so the classical prosthetic valve sounds are lost.
- If a woman presents unwell and a new murmur is heard, endocarditis (Chapter 6) should be excluded.

Investigation

- Similar to that of the native valve (see Chapter 5).
- Trans-thoracic echo may be a little less clear due to artefact of the prosthesis and a trans-oesophageal echo may be required if there is concern about endocarditis.

Pregnancy management

The effect of the pregnancy on patients' post valve surgery

- The majority of problems in women post valve surgery are in those with prosthetic heart valves.
- Whilst anticoagulation (See Chapter 17) poses the commonest difficulty in pregnancy, prosthetic heart valves are associated with a number of other complications:
  - thromboembolism
  - structural failure
  - infection.
- In the well-managed non-pregnant woman, the overall annual incidence of complications is approximately 3%.
- Relative risk of death from mechanical valves is double that of biological valves with overall risk of 1–2%.
- In one study of valve replacements in pregnancy, valve loss at 10 years was higher with bioprosthetic valves (82%) than mechanical (29%) or homografts (28%).

Ross procedure for aortic valve disease

- Operation to move native pulmonary valve to aortic position (pulmonary autograft) and insert bioprosthetic valve in low pressure pulmonary position in attempt to improve longevity of bioprosthetic valve.
- Two studies have found no evidence of pregnancy related structural deterioration whilst a third found that homografts were associated with less reoperation when compared to bioprosthetic valves.
- It may be therefore that the Ross procedure will be the preferred valve operation of choice in young women requiring aortic valve surgery.

Complications of previous valve surgery

Valve thrombosis

Risk factors

- Older valves, e.g. 'ball and cage' Starr Edwards valve.
- Smaller valves (this may be highly relevant in women who had surgery at a young age before reaching full adult size).
- Valves in the mitral position.
- Women with multiple valves.
- Women with previous history of valve thrombosis or embolic events.

Diagnosis

- Valve thrombosis should be considered in women with unexpected dyspnoea.
- Valves often stick half closed or half open hence are often not associated with sudden cardiac death.
- Clear metallic sounds are lost on ausculatation.
- Confirmation is with either.
  - echo
  - flouroscopic valve screening.

Treatment

- Thrombolysis
  - Risk of retroplacental haemorrhage and fetal loss
- Surgery
  - As risky as thrombolysis for fetus and high risk for mother.

Development of new or worsening valve lesion in pregnancy

- This is most commonly found in women with previous mitral valve surgery who develop aortic disease really?
- Usually no worse than moderate.
- Individual lesions should be managed as discussed in valve chapter.

Prosthetic valve dysfunction

- Valve thrombosis (discussed above).
- Increasing regurgitation during pregnancy.
- Infective endocarditis should be considered in sudden dysfunction.

Impaired ventricular function

- Some patients who have undergone previous valve surgery have impaired LV or RV function.
- This is associated with increased morbidity and mortality, as discussed in Chapter 22.

The effects of valve replacement on the fetus

- Women with a prosthetic heart valve have a higher rate of fetal morbidity and mortality than normal pregnancies.
- Stillbirths range between 2 and 8%.
- Some groups have reported a miscarriage rate up to 23% (majority in women on anticoagulant therapy).
- Between 70 and 85% of pregnancies result in a successful outcome although the preterm delivery rate is higher and there is no difference between those babies born to mothers with bioprosthetic valves compared to mechanical valves.

Pre-pregnancy counselling

Increasing numbers of women of child-bearing age have undergone previous valvular surgical intervention.

It is imperative that women are counselled prior to conception to allow them to understand the risks both to themselves and the fetus of undergoing a pregnancy so couples can make an informed decision as to whether they want to proceed.

Areas of particular concern are:

- Drugs in pregnancy:
  - warfarin – this is discussed fully in Chapter 17
  - women may be taking other teratogenic drugs, e.g. ACE inhibitors, etc. which are required for the on-going well-being of the mother.
- Life expectancy:
  - whilst many women have a long life-expectancy with corrected valvular heart disease, when counselling women and their partners it is important to take into account the expected natural history of the condition
  - this is particularly important in women with impaired left ventricular function
  - the risk of maternal death is approximately 7% if the patient is in New York Heart Association (NYHA) class III or IV.
- Valve deterioration:
  - bioprostheses have limited durability – pregnancy may accelerate valve deterioration.
- Timing of pregnancy:
  - it is important to understand the natural history of the valve and patients condition and advise re optimum time to undergo a pregnancy
  - if considering first pregnancy, fertility issues may not yet have come to light, especially in the older primagravida, i.e. it may take many years to conceive
  - it is probably sensible to recommend a woman waits at least 1 year post surgery to allow full post-operative recovery, particularly of the sternum, before conceiving.

Contraception in prosthetic valves

See Chapter 23.

Intrauterine contraceptive devices (Copper IUCDs)

- Are associated with a significant risk of menorrhagia (35%) in patients having undergone cardiac surgery, predominantly due to anticoagulant therapy.
- Possible endocarditis risk.
- Therefore probably best avoided.

Barrier methods

- Unreliable.

The combined (oestrogen and progesterone) oral contraceptive pill

- Contraindicated in women with pre-existing hypertension, thromboembolic disorders, cerebrovascular disease, and coronary artery disease.

Progesterone based contraception

- **Preferred method of contraception**, e.g. Mirena®, Implanon® or Cerazette®. Mirena intrauterine system (IUS) is also a coil; however, it releases a progesterone making it more effective and is not metal therefore does not carry the endocarditis risk of standard copper IUCDs.

Delivery and the puerperium

- For most cardiac conditions a normal vaginal delivery with good analgesia and a low threshold for mechanical assistance is the safest mode of delivery for the mother, as it is associated with less blood loss, reduced risk of haemorrhage, thrombosis and infection, and reduced rapid haemodynamic changes compared to caesarean section.
- Women with an older generation mechanical (e.g. Bjork-Shiley) mitral valve may be considered for elective caesarean section to reduce the time off anticoagulation, though this is controversial.
- Despite the risks of endocarditis particularly around the time of delivery, the incidence of prosthetic valve endocarditis appears to be low (see Chapter 6).

Conclusion

With the appropriate intensive multidisciplinary care, the outcome of women who have undergone cardiac valve replacement surgery is favourable, providing their underlying left ventricular function is good.

Cardiac surgery in pregnancy

Cardiac surgery in pregnancy

Cardiac surgery in pregnancy is rare and only undertaken when medical therapy fails and percutaneous treatment is unavailable or unsuitable.

Cardiac bypass surgery is associated with a high risk to the fetus (20–33% risk of fetal death) however the literature is divided about maternal risk.

In some series maternal risk is similar to that for the non-pregnant woman (3% overall) however many papers state a risk around 10–15%. This is likely to reflect the fact that most procedures in pregnancy are emergencies. Increased mortality is associated with:
- emergency procedures
- maternal haemodynamic instability and co-morbidity
- aortic surgery (e.g. dissection) and pulmonary embolectomy (22% compared to 9% for valvular operations)
- surgery at the time of delivery or immediately post-partum
- early gestational age.

Morbidity is high in those who survive with one quarter of mothers having significant sequelae post operatively and 10% of fetuses severely affected.

Risks

Risks from surgery are due to a combination of:
- need for anticoagulation
- cooling during surgery
- the effect of removing normal pulsatile flow to the uterus whilst on bypass
- anaesthetic agents.

Cardiopulmonary bypass can lead to a fetal bradycardia related to hypoperfusion.

As neonatal services are much improved, Caesarean section early in the third trimester immediately before commencing cardiopulmonary bypass may be a better option for a favourable outcome for both mother and fetus.
- Prior to 23 weeks the fetus is not considered viable and so the woman should be counselled about possible fetal demise.
- After 28 weeks it is probably preferable to deliver the baby before cardiac bypass surgery.
- Between 24–28 weeks a decision will need to made on an individual basis, after thorough counselling of the mother, regarding the risks of fetal distress during the procedure and the impracticalities of monitoring the baby during cardiac surgery and performing an emergency delivery in this situation.

Methods to improve fetal outcomes

Methods to improve fetal outcomes include:
- high flow, high pressure normothermic bypass
- using pulsatile flow
- intraoperative external fetal heart monitoring during surgery but this is usually impractical
- uterine monitoring to assess contractions
- administration of beta-2 agonists or other tocolytics to prevent uterine contractions
- pre-operative administration of steroids to induce fetal lung maturation in the event of the need for urgent delivery.

If surgery can be withheld in pregnancy, deciding the optimal time to operate on the post-natal women is also difficult. Risks remains high post partum and whilst there is no consensus on the optimum time for surgery post-partum, it is best delayed until at least 3 months post-partum if the clinical situation allows.

Arrhythmias

Introduction

Incidence of arrhythmias in pregnancy

- Palpitations in pregnancy are common.
- Cardiac arrhythmias can be identified on Holter recordings in up to 60% of normal people under the age of 40.
- Ectopic beats and non-sustained arrhythmias occur in more than 50% of pregnant women investigated for palpitations.
- Sustained tachycardias however occur in only 2–3/1000 of such women.

Presentation

- Presentation can either be as a recurrence of a previously known arrhythmia or first presentation in pregnancy.
- The majority of arrhythmias are benign requiring only reassurance.
- In the remaining minority of cases, judicious use of anti-arrhythmic drugs usually leads to a safe and successful outcome for both mother and baby.
- There were no documented maternal deaths from primary arrhythmias in the last confidential enquiry into maternal mortality, but 6% of cardiac deaths were defined as sudden adult death syndrome, which raises the possibility of death from a primary arrhythmia.

The mechanism of arrhythmia

- The combination of the adaptive changes to pregnancy, e.g. ↑ HR and CO (see Chapter 1 Physiological changes in pregnancy) and the heightened visceral awareness experienced in pregnancy may lead a woman to seek advice on symptoms that are within the normal range and may otherwise have been ignored.
- The pregnant state is unlikely to generate a new arrhythmia substrate; however, such physiological changes may render a pre-existing substrate capable of sustaining an arrhythmia.
- Many tachycardias are initiated by ectopic beats which are known to increase in pregnancy.

Table 9.1 Mechanism of arrhythmia generation

Structural heart disease	Structurally normal heart
Congenital heart disease creating re-entrant circuits	**Congenital 'electrical only' disease**
Acyanotic heart disease, e.g. ASD/VSD	Dual AV nodal pathways causing AVNRT
Cyanotic heart disease, e.g. Fallots	WPW/accessory pathway
Valvular heart disease, e.g. bicuspid aortic valve	'Channelopathy'
Acquired	**Acquired**
Valvular heart disease 2° to rheumatic fever	**Degenerative disease of conduction system**
Valvular heart disease 2° to endocarditis	Acquired Long QT syndrome, e.g. drugs, metabolic
Cardiomyopathy	

Reproduced with permission from Lefoy and Adamson (2007) Heart Rhythm Disorders. In: Oakley and Warnes, eds. *Heart Disease in Pregnancy*. Wiley–Blackwell.

Diagnosis of arrhythmia

1. Obtain accurate diagnosis to give reliable advice regarding treatment and prognosis.
2. Determine whether there is additional heart disease associated with the arrhythmia, e.g. MV disease.
3. Exclude systemic disorders that present with arrhythmias, e.g. thyrotoxicosis, pulmonary embolus (PE).

History

- In late pregnancy, minor arrhythmias may present with breathlessness and chest pain.
- Syncope may simply be from physiological drop in BP, which is maximum in the 2nd trimester.
- Thorough family history for sudden premature or unexplained deaths to identify genetic propensity to life threatening arrhythmias.
- Women with previous atrial surgery or with RV impairment are prone to arrhythmias especially atrial flutter.

Investigations modalities used in arrhythmia diagnosis

(See Table 9.2)

- Attempt to record 12 lead ECG during arrhythmia.
- Holter or event monitors can be very useful for frequent arrhythmias, but a symptom diary should be kept.
- Asymptomatic arrhythmias should not be treated unless they are felt to be life threatening.
- There is no evidence of implantable loop recorders having been used in pregnancy but there are no theoretical reasons why they cannot be used.

Table 9.2 Diagnostic modalities used in arrhythmia diagnosis

Echocardiogram	This should be considered an integral part of the investigation of any pregnant patient with proven arrhythmia to diagnose structural and functional heart disease.
Exercise ECG	This can be reasonably carried out during pregnancy providing exercise is not contraindicated for obstetric reasons. Care should be taken not to exceed the woman's normal exercise capability and the test should be stopped if hypotension develops as this may impair placental perfusion.
Tilt-table testing	Whilst there has been experience of this in pregnancy, it is usually possible to delay this investigation until after pregnancy. It is also difficult to do beyond 24 weeks as women are unable to lie flat on their backs as the gravid uterus impedes IVC flow.
Pharmacological testing	A pharmacological challenge may provide important diagnostic information particularly in narrow complex tachycardia. Adenosine has been widely used in pregnancy, though predominantly for arrhythmia termination. There is no reported experience of Ajmaline or flecainide challenge for Brugada syndrome in pregnancy. Flecainide has safely been used in pregnancy.
Electrophysiological studies	This is rarely required in pregnancy as the arrhythmia can usually be managed pharmacologically until after delivery.

Anti-arrhythmic drugs

The decision to treat a woman depends upon the following:
- frequency of arrhythmia
- duration of arrhythmia
- tolerability of the arrhythmia
- it is a balance between arrhythmia reduction or termination *versus* maternal and fetal side-effects of drug therapy:
  - the greatest risk to the fetus is during the 1st trimester, i.e. during organogenesis
  - the smallest dose should be used and maternal and fetal monitoring should be carried out.

NB: Patients may have break through arrhythmias in pregnancy due to reductions in therapeutic drug levels due to the changing volume of distribution and drug metabolism.

Table 9.3 details those anti-arrhythmics which are safe to use in pregnancy. The majority of drugs, however, only have class C evidence for their use.

Beta-blockers in pregnancy
- There is historic concern over beta-blockers in pregnancy and FGR (fetal growth restriction).
- This effect now appears to be limited to atenolol when used during the 1st trimester.
- FGR is not seen when other beta blockers are used in the 1st trimester or if atenolol is taken in the 2nd or 3rd trimester only.

When benefit exceeds risk, as in the following conditions, beta blockers should not be withheld. In such circumstances, 4-weekly fetal growth scans from 24 to 26 weeks are recommended.
- Significant arrhythmias.
- Mitral stenosis.
- Marfans syndrome.
- Thyrotoxicosis.

See p. 91 for use of beta-blockers in AF/Aflutter and MS (Chapter 5 native valves section).

DC cardioversion

- Appears safe in all stages of pregnancy.
- Amount of current reaching fetus small due to amniotic fluid therefore very small risk of causing fetal arrhythmias.
- Fetus should be monitored throughout procedure.
- Consult with an obstetric anaesthetist re optimal sedation/anaesthesia because of risk of aspiration.
- Women should be placed in left lateral position to move gravid uterus off vena cava.
- Procedure otherwise same as for non-pregnant women.

Implantable defibrillators (see Figure 9.1)

- Women with automatic implantable cardiac defibrillators (AICDs) have successfully negotiated pregnancy with good fetal outcomes.
- Theoretical risk of defibrillator thresholds changing in pregnancy.
- Studies appear to show no increase in either device or therapy complications nor any increase in the number of shocks the women received compared to pre-conception.
- Monitoring of the baby with a cardiotocogram to ensure satisfactory fetal well-being must be considered after each therapy episode.
- For those pregnant women with on-going malignant arrhythmias despite pharmacological therapy, an ICD may be a safe alternative.
- Theoretical concern with unipolar diathermy if caesarean section required.
- Recommend disarming (magnet can be used for emergency caesarean section) during caesarean section then checking device post natally
- If a magnet is placed over the patient's device will turn off any therapy modalities on the device and revert it to a pacemaker only. This will prevent any interference to be misread as an arrhythmia.
- If VT/VF does occur during caesarean section, the magnet can simply be removed to allow device to fire.

Table 9.3 Anti-arrhythmic drugs

Drugs	Safety profile	Listed complications	Breast feeding
Adenosine	Safe to use in pregnancy with no detectable effect on fetal cardiac rhythm	Pregnant women may respond to lower doses due to a reduction in adenosine deaminase	Safe as short half life
Atropine	Unknown but has been used for resuscitation	Insufficient data	Unknown
Amiodarone	Only for short term use in emergencies	If prolonged use; fetal hypo- & hyper thyroidism, goitre, FGR, prematurity	Avoid
Beta-blockers	Avoid atenolol in first trimester unless no suitable alternative because of concern over FGR	FGR, bradycardia, apnoea, hypoglycaemia hyperbilirubinaemia are all rare	Safe
Digoxin	Good safety profile	Miscarriage & fetal death in toxicity	Safe
Diltiazem	Too little experience to comment	Skeletal abnormalities, FGR, fetal death	Unknown
Disopyramide	Too little data to recommend regular use	Premature uterine contractions	Unknown
Flecainide	Limited literature for treatment of maternal arrhythmias however maternal ingestion is used to treat fetal SVT	Insufficient data but no reported significant complications. Concerns over its pro-arrhythmic potential in fetus have limited its use in past	Unknown
Lignocaine	Good	Fetal distress may occur in fetal toxicity	Safe
Quinidine	Good safety profile in pregnancy however not used because of concern over safety profile in non-pregnant women	Rarely; mild uterine contractions, premature labour, neonatal thrombocytopenia, fetal VIII cranial nerve damage	Safe
Procainamide	Possibly as safe as quinidine short term in pregnancy	Chronic use may be associated with lupus like syndrome, GI disturbance, hypotension, agranulocytosis	Safe

Table 9.3 (*Contd.*) Anti-arrhythmic drugs

Drugs	Safety profile	Listed complications	Breast feeding
Propafenone	Unknown	Insufficient data	Unknown
Sotalol	Safe	Transient fetal bradycardia	Safe
Verapamil	Safe (1st choice class IV drug)	Rapid injection may cause maternal ↓ BP and fetal distress	Safe

FGR = fetal growth retardation

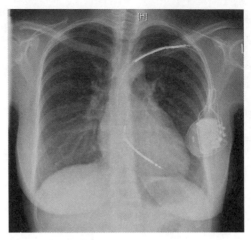

Fig. 9.1 CXR of patient with implantable defibrillator.

Termination of specific arrhythmias

Bradycardia in pregnancy

- Pathological bradycardia in pregnant women is rare.
- Rarely, symptomatic bradycardia has been attributed to supine hypotensive syndrome of pregnancy, which is a result of compression of the inferior vena cava by the gravid uterus and responds to maternal changing of position.
- Congenital heart block (CHB) is rare and does not usually pose a problem during the pregnancy.
- Temporary pacing wire is usually not required during delivery.
- Spinal anaesthesia for caesarean section (CS) can be associated with a higher incidence of all grades of bradycardia (up to 13%).
- In the rare cases of a pregnant woman requiring a permanent pacemaker (PPM), try and avoid inserting in the first trimester and use minimal radiation.

Supraventicular tacycardia (SVT) **(Figure 9.2)**

- Drug choice is dependent upon SVT being treated.
- Patients should be taught vagotonic manoeuvres as first therapy.
- Adenosine is safe to use in pregnancy—most women respond to between 6 and 12 mg.
- Verapamil is an effective second line treatment for the treatment of SVTs and can be used in doses up to 10 mg without affecting fetal heart rate.
- Fetal distress has been associated with verapamil induced maternal hypotension.
- Beta-blockers are the drugs of choice in women with known WPW, as AV nodal blocking drugs may accelerate conduction through the accessory pathway and cause deterioration in maternal condition.

Atrial fibrillation and flutter **(Figure 9.3—AF, Figure 9.4—a flutter)**

- These arrhythmias are uncommon in pregnancy.
- If seen, they are most commonly associated with congenital or valvular heart disease as well as metabolic disturbances such as thyrotoxicosis, electrolyte disturbance, systemic illness such as infection, or pulmonary embolus.
- Though often well tolerated (apart from in severe mitral stenosis), it is advantageous to terminate the arrhythmia to avoid the need for anti-coagulation, particularly as pregnancy is a pro-thrombotic state.
- Preferred drugs for arrhythmia termination/rate control:
  - beta-blockers, e.g. sotalol, atenolol
  - digoxin (for rate control only)
  - verapamil
  - flecainide
  - procainamide
  - amiodarone has been used in acute setting.

- Women need to be anti-coagulated as soon as possible initially with LMWH until arrhythmia terminated (see Chapter 17).
- Best to restore sinus rhythm where possible both for improved cardiac output as well as to avoid the need for anticoagulation.

Atrial fibrillation/flutter in mitral stenosis (MS)

- In MS, ventricular filling is reduced.
- Ventricular filling is reduced further with the high rates associated with AF/flutter due to a reduction in time for diastole.
- This causes increased filling pressures.
- This process may rapidly degenerate into pulmonary oedema.
- This requires usual treatment, i.e. oxygen, diuretics, nitrates etc however a beta-blocker to reduce heart rate (IV if neccessary) may be life saving in this situation.

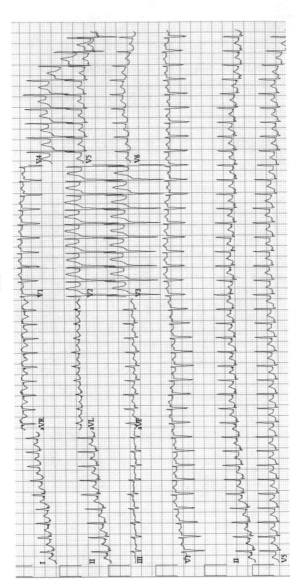

Fig. 9.2 ECG of supraventricular tachycardia at rate of 240. This is a AVNRT due to conduction down an accessory pathway.

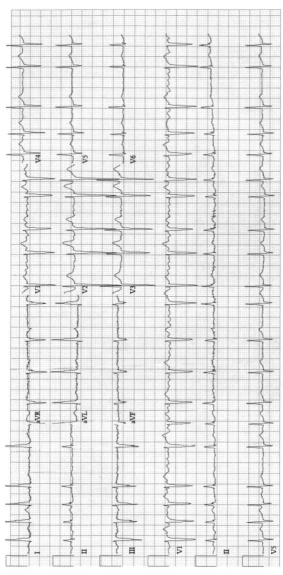

Fig. 9.3 ECG of atrial fibrillation. There is an irregular rhythm with absence of "p" waves.

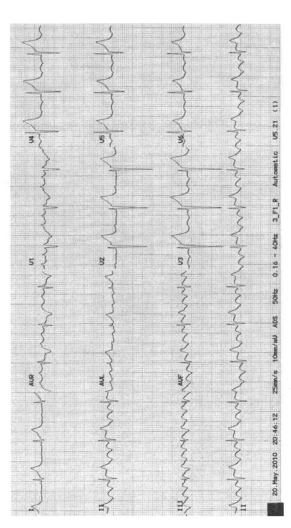

Fig. 9.4 ECG of atrial flutter. The classical 'saw tooth' atrial activity can be clearly seen in leads III and aVF.

VT in the structurally abnormal heart

- Any disease process that affects the ventricular myocardium causing scarring, hypertrophy, or infiltration may disrupt the electrical integrity of the myocardium.
- Rapid VT causes hypotension, reduced myocardial coronary perfusion, and subendocardial ischaemia, an unstable situation that may degenerate into ventricular fibrillation.
- VT in the presence of structural heart disease is associated with a significant risk of sudden death and requires emergency treatment.
- Treatment should be with IV lignocaine, amiodarone, or DC cardioversion.
- Amiodarone is best reserved for use in emergency situation as it can affect the fetal thyroid. However, if required due to malignant arrhythmia in the mother, do not withhold.

Polymorphic VT (Torsade de point) **(Figure 9.5)**

- Unless polymorphic VT spontaneously terminates within a few seconds, it invariably causes collapse and has a high risk of degenerating into ventricular fibrillation.

The emergency treatment requires:
- Correction of electrolyte disturbance including magnesium.
- Removal of precipitating drugs, particularly:
  - class I and III antiarrhythmic drugs
  - macrolide antibiotics, e.g. erythromycin
  - non-sedating antihistamines
  - antidepressants
  - antipsychotics.
- Consider temporary overdrive pacing.

VT in the structurally normal heart (Idiopathic VT) **(Figure 9.6)**

- This is the most common form of VT seen in pregnancy.
- It virtually never accelerates to an unstable rhythm
- If QRS morphology LBBB, responds to beta-blockers – most common form.
- If QRS morphology RBBB, responds well to verapamil (less common).

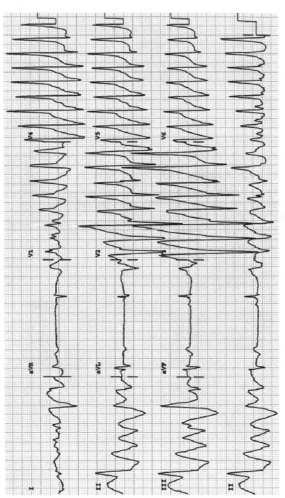

Fig. 9.5 This ECG demonstrates polymorphic ventricular tachycardia (torsades de point).

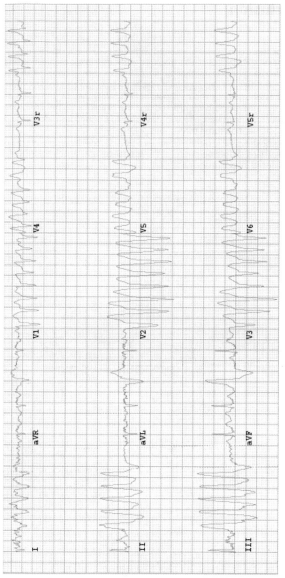

Fig. 9.6 This ECG is taken from a young pregnant woman and shows self terminating runs of a broad complex tachycardia which originates from the right ventricular outflow tract (RVOT). This the most common form of VT in the structurally normal heart.

Conclusion

Management of arrhythmias should ideally start before conception, but during pregnancy, medication should only be initiated if symptoms are severe or the arrhythmia is associated with haemodynamic compromise.

In general arrhythmias can be managed without specific medication and with little risk to either mother or fetus. Reassurance is often all that is required. If drugs are required then ideally they should be avoided in the first trimester and drug choice should reflect safety data in pregnancy as well as the arrhythmia being treated and the presence of any structural heart disease. The lowest effective dose should be used and mother and fetus should be monitored throughout pregnancy.

In emergencies, DC cardioversion is safe and whilst cardiac arrest is rare, physicians should be aware of the special circumstances that should be considered in its management.

Cardiomyopathies

Cardiomyopathies

- Cardiomyopathy is the cause of almost a quarter of cardiac maternal deaths
- Dilated cardiomyopathy (DCM), hypertrophic cardiomyopathy (HCM), and restrictive cardiomyopathy usually predate the pregnancy but may first present in pregnancy
- Peripartum cardiomyopathy (PPCM) is specific to pregnancy.

Peripartum cardiomyopathy (PPCM)

Definition
- Onset of heart failure with no identifiable cause in the absence of heart disease occurring between the last month of pregnancy and the first 5 months post-partum
- Rare: incidence 1:5000 to 1:10000
- Similar in its clinical presentation to dilated cardiomyopathy (DCM), but the latter is not related to pregnancy and patients with DCM are usually older.

Aetiology
Unknown, although theories include:
- viral antigen persistence and virus-associated inflammatory changes
- cardiac myocyte apoptosis
- microchimerism
- autoimmune and genetic factors
- hormonal – excessive prolactin production.

Risk factors
- Increased maternal age.
- Afrocaribbean race.
- Multiparity.
- Multiple pregnancy.
- Hypertension (pre-existing, pregnancy induced or pre-eclampsia).

Clinical
- Presentation varies from an incidental finding during echocardiography through to severe heart failure and death.
- The symptoms may be difficult to differentiate from the normal signs and symptoms of pregnancy, particularly in women in the last trimester.
- Women typically present with shortness of breath, orthopnoea, paroxsmal nocturnal dyspnoea, or features of right heart failure with marked oedema.
- May have cough and wheeze (often initially misdiagnosed as asthma), palpitations, and embolic phenomena (pulmonary embolus/systemic emboli from mural thrombus).

Examination
- Tachycardia often with gallop rhythm, tachypnoea, wheeze, congestive cardiac failure +/− arrhythmia.
- Cardiac decompensation in an otherwise stable patient may occur with fluid overload which can be caused by:
  • Iatrogenic fluid infusions
  • syntocinon infusions
  • β-agonists for tocolysis
  • steroids for fetal lung maturity.

Investigations

- CXR: enlarged heart and pulmonary congestion/pulmonary oedema +/− bilateral pleural effusions (see Figure 10.1).
- ECG: tachycardia +/− atrial or ventricular arrhythmias.
- Echocardiography: usually global dilatation, often of all four chambers of the heart. Specifically:
  - left ventricular ejection fraction (LVEF) <45%
  - fractional shortening < 30%
  - left ventricular end-diastolic dimension (LVEDD) > 2.7cm/m^2.

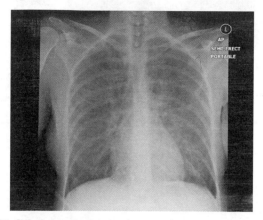

Fig. 10.1 CXR of pregnant woman in pulmonary oedema.

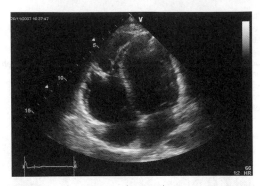

Fig. 10.2 Echo image of peripartum cardiomyopathy.

Complications

Maternal
- Systemic or pulmonary emboli from mural thrombus.
- Fatal arrhythmias.
- Death.

Fetal
- Preterm delivery (usually iatrogenic) and associated morbidity.
- Death.

Diagnosis

This is made by a combination of:
- a temporal relationship with pregnancy and
- echocardiography findings and
- exclusion of other causes of heart failure.

Differential diagnosis

- Dilated cardiomyopathy of a different aetiology, e.g. idiopathic DCM, viral myocarditis.
- Pulmonary thrombo-embolism.
- Myocardial infarction.

Treatment
- Multidisciplinary involvement if still pregnant or within 6 weeks of delivery with:
  - Cardiologist
  - Obstetric physician (if available)
  - Obstetrician (maternal medicine specialist)
  - Obstetric anaesthetist
- Pulmonary oedema: oxygen and loop diuretics.
- Reduce afterload: with vasodilators
  - *Antenatally*:
    — nifedipine, hydralazine or isosorbide
    — cardioselective beta blockers—e.g. bisoprolol
    — diuretics but caution in women with associated pre-eclampsia.
  - *Postnatally*:
    — nifedipine, hydralazine or isosorbide
    — cardioselective beta blockers—e.g. bisoprolol
    — diuretics but caution in women with associated pre-eclampsia
    — ACE inhibitors, e.g. enalapril.
- Thromboprophylaxis:
  - LMWH high prophylactic dose, e.g. enoxaparin (Clexane®) 40 mg bd
  - higher dose LMWH if obese
  - full anticoagulation doses of LMWH if associated arrhythmias or embolic phenomena
  - if full anticoagulation required postnatally e.g. arrhythmias, use warfarin (safe in breast feeding).
- Anti-arrhythmics:
  - atrial fibrillation or flutter: digoxin and flecainide safe
  - rate control in those with preserved cardiac output can use cardioselective β-blockers with caution.
- If remains hypoxic and hypotensive:
  - intubate and ventilate
  - inotropic support
  - if antenatal, deliver fetus by caesarean to facilitate reduction in cardiac workload.
  - close liaison with cardiac transplant centre
  - may need an intra-aortic balloon pump or a left ventricular assist device as a bridge to myocardial recovery or cardiac transplantation.

Delivery
- Delivery should be expedited if PPCM is diagnosed antenatally. This may result in iatrogenic preterm delivery.
- If steroids for fetal lung maturation are required (if gestation <34–36 weeks), cover with diuretics to avoid fluid overload.

Vaginal delivery
- Appropriate if relatively mild disease or if adequately treated.
- Invasive monitoring in labour with arterial and central venous lines.
- Pulmonary wedge readings not usually necessary.
- Treat increase in central venous pressure (CVP) with diuretics.
- Treat tachycardia with intravenous β-blockers, e.g. metoprolol.
- Recommend early regional analgesia (assists pain control and prevention of maternal tachycardia) – consultant anaesthetic involvement imperative.

Induction of labour (IOL)
- Allows all relevant senior staff to be available for labour and delivery and insertion of lines.
- if receiving twice daily LMWH preparations, IOL allows the heparin dose to be omitted prior to the onset of labour, thereby allowing the use of regional anaesthesia.

Caesarean section
- Should ideally be used for obstetric indications only.
- If significant maternal compromise with severe disease then it may be necessary.
- If required, aim to carry out in conjunction with cardiothoracic anaesthetist.
- General anaesthesia may be necessary if the woman is unable to lie almost flat (see Chapter 26).

Third stage
- Dilute infusion of 5 units of syntocinon to prevent maternal tachycardia and hypotension with bolus syntocinon.

Post-partum haemorrhage
- Medical management: use ergometrine, misoprostol. Can use syntocinon infusion.
- Surgical methods may be necessary: e.g. intrauterine balloon, B-Lynch or Brace suture (see Chapter 24).

Post-partum
- Continue thromboprophylaxis if no bleeding concerns.
- Add ACE inhibitor (can breast feed): This should be continued at least until LV function returns to normal.
- Re-echo 6 months after discontinuing ACE to ensure LV still normal off treatment.

Prognosis
- Maternal mortality:
  - poor NYHA functional class is a predictor of mortality
  - maternal mortality rate from PPCM declining: recent studies suggest 9–15%
  - the deaths that occur are usually within a few months of diagnosis.

- 30–50% improve with treatment and return to normal.
  - more likely if LVEF >30% at diagnosis
  - usually recovered within 6 months of diagnosis.
- Others improve slowly and are left with a degree of LV impairment.
  - may improve over years or
  - may deteriorate despite full medical intervention and require heart transplant
  - poor long-term prognosis related to degree of LV dysfunction at diagnosis and larger LV diameters.

Subsequent pregnancy

- Pre-pregnancy counselling imperative: discuss risk of cardiac decompensation and maternal death.

Persistent LV dysfunction or dilatation 6 months after initial diagnosis of PPCM

- Pregnancy not advised.
- If conceives:
  - 50% risk of worsening cardiac failure
  - 42% risk of persistent fall in LVEF of >20%
  - 25% risk maternal death.
- Recommend effective contraception, e.g. intra-uterine progestogen-only system (Mirena®) or subdermal progestogen-only implant (Implanon®).
- Offer termination of pregnancy.

LV function returned to normal

- If conceives:
  - 26% risk of cardiac failure
  - 9% risk of persistent fall in LVEF of >20%
- Likely that those with reduced contractile reserve may decompensate with haemodynamic stress of a future pregnancy.
- Prenatal exercise or dobutaine stress echocardiography may help identify those with reduced contractile reserve but the data are currently limited.

If subsequent pregnancy

- Re-assess and counsel again regarding risks.
- If unplanned pregnancy consider termination of pregnancy if persistent LV dysfunction.
- Baseline echocardiogram and repeat echocardiogram at regular intervals.
- Full hospital combined obstetric and cardiology care.
- Stop teratogenic medications and replace as necessary.
- If clinical or echocardiographic deterioration, serious consideration should be given to discontinuation of the pregnancy either as a termination of pregnancy or preterm delivery.

Dilated cardiomyopathies (DCM)

- Congestive cardiac failure secondary to dilatation and systolic (and/or diastolic) dysfunction of the ventricle(s).
- Left ventricle usually affected.
- May be related to other conditions (see Table 10.1) or no known cause (idiopathic DCM).

Table 10.1 Causes of dilated cardiomyopathy

Group	Examples
Infections	Viral: coxsackie B, HIV, Ebstein-Barr virus, varicella, echovirus, measles, mumps, rubella, polio TB, rickettsia, parasites, fungi
Connective tissue diseases	Systemic lupus erythematosus, rheumatoid arthritis, dermatomyositis
Haematological	Sickle cell disease, thalassaemia, iron deficiency anaemia
Endocrine	Hypo- and hyperthyroidism, hypoparathyroidism, pheochromocytoma
Drugs	Alcohol, chloroquine, iron overload, cyclophosphamide
Nutritional deficiencies	Niacin, thiamine, selenium deficiencies, Kwashiorkor
Vascular	Kawasaki disease
Cardiac	Ischaemic heart disease, arrhythmogenic right ventricular cardiomyopathy
Muscular	Muscular dystrophies
Metabolic	Hemochromatosis, glycogen storage disorders, fatty acid oxidation defects, carnitine deficiency

Diagnostic criteria

- LVEF < 45% and/or.
- Fractional shortening <25% and.
- LVEDD > 112% predicted for age and body surface area.

Echocardiography

- All four cardiac chambers dilated.
- LV affected more often than RV.
- Varying degrees of functional mitral and tricuspid regurgitation due to dilated valve rings.
- Mural thrombus may occur at LV apex in severely affected ventricles or within the atria.

Pathogenesis of myocardial damage
- Infective myocarditis.
- Autoimmunity.
- Genetic predisposition.

Pregnancy
- Pregnancy with impaired LV function from any cause can result in further deterioration in LV function with inability to meet the demands of an increased cardiac output.
- Pregnancy not advised if severely impaired LV function.
- Termination of pregnancy may be necessary.
- Otherwise manage as for PPCM.

Predictors of adverse events
- New York Heart Association (NYHA) grade 3–4.
- Left Ventricular Ejection Fraction (LVEF) <30%.

Prognosis
- Idiopathic DCM outside pregnancy, 3-year survival
  - 92% if ejection fraction >40%
  - 71% if ejection fraction <30%.
- Few data in pregnancy.

Hypertrophic cardiomyopathy (HCM)

In some patients, the hypertrophy can cause outflow tract obstruction in which case the condition is known as Hypertrophic obstructive cardiomyopthy (HOCM) however it is important to understand that it is all a spectrum of the same condition.

Incidence
- 1:2000.
- 70% autosomal dominant inheritance.

Diagnosis
- Usually following echocardiography to investigate symptoms, heart murmur or positive family history.
- Unexplained asymmetrical ventricular hypertrophy on echocardiography.
- Maximal wall thickness exceeding 2 standard deviations for age.

Clinical features
- Often asymptomatic.
- Chest pain.
- Breathlessness.
- Pre-syncope, syncope (due to obstruction of LV outflow tract).
- Arrythmias (atrial or ventricular).
- Heart failure.
- Sudden death.

Complications
Overall risk of disease related complications (sudden death, end-stage heart failure, stroke) = 1–2% per year.

Sudden death
- Most sudden deaths occur with LV wall thickness <3 mm
- Risk factors for sudden death:
  - family history: ≥2 sudden cardiac deaths in <40 years old
  - failure of BP to rise >25 mmHg from baseline following exercise
  - ventricular tachycardia.
- Can occur in pregnancy reflecting background expected rate.

Pregnancy and HCM
- Small risk of symptoms developing in asymptomatic women.
- 10–40% of women symptomatic pre-pregnancy deteriorate in pregnancy.
- May not tolerate tachycardia, reduction in preload, or reduction in afterload.
- May develop pulmonary oedema due to diastolic dysfunction.

Management in pregnancy
• If symptomatic reduce heart rate with β-blockers.
• Treat any arrhythmias (see Chapter 9).
• If asymptomatic can deliver in local unit, otherwise deliver in a tertiary unit with a multidisciplinary team.
• Aim for vaginal delivery.
• Caesarean section for obstetric indications or if decompensated.
• Care with regional analgesia and anaesthesia which causes peripheral dilatation and reduction in afterload. Preload with fluid prior to insertion.
• Hypovolaemia will reduce preload.
• Keep well-filled during labour and delivery.
• Ensure rapid fluid resuscitation following any antepartum or post-partum haemorrhage.

A significant number of patients may have an automatic implantable cardiac defibrillator (AICD) inserted for primary or secondary prevention of life threatening ventricular arrhythmias or sudden cardiac death. The management of this is discussed in Chapter 8.

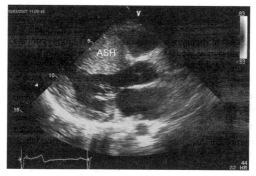

Fig. 10.3 Parasternal long axis of a 19-yr-old girl with marked asymmetrical septal hypertrophy (ASH), one of the markers of hypertrophic cardiomyopathy.

Cardiac transplantation

Main indication postnatally is peripartum cardiomyopathy, but in most women who present in pregnancy having had cardiac transplantation it is for causes unrelated to pregnancy.

Pregnancy following cardiac transplantation

- Increasing cases reported as more adult cardiac transplantation occurring and paediatric cardiac transplant recipient population surviving to childbearing age.
- Women are usually fertile and require pre-pregnancy counselling and/or adequate contraception.
- Immunosuppression must continue in pregnancy to prevent transplant rejection.
- Previous pregnancy increases risk of rejection.
- Vast experience of immunosuppressive agents from pregnant renal transplant patients. Combinations of prednisolone, azathioprine and cyclosporine routinely used. Increasing data on MMF use in pregnancy: teratogenic and usually switched to azathioprine pre pregnancy.
- Often successful outcomes with similar risks to renal and liver transplant patients.
- Maternal risks:
  - pregnancy-induced hypertension
  - pre-eclampsia
  - renal insufficiency (related to CNI—[calcineurin inhibitor], e.g. ciclosporin) use
  - although theoretically PPCM can recur, no reported cases of recurrence in cardiac transplant recipients who go on to conceive
  - patients with cardiac transplants also develop premature coronary artery disease.
- Fetal risks:
  - prematurity
  - low birth weight.
- Vaginal delivery appropriate unless obstetric indication for caesarean section.

Chapter 11

151

Pulmonary hypertension

Pulmonary hypertension (PHT)

- Pregnancy is contraindicated in PHT
- Disease modifying drugs, are allowing women diagnosed with PHT to live longer and with less symptoms, and so these women are starting to attempt pregnancy
- Increasing experience is being gained and some women have had successful outcomes BUT as mortality remains extremely high (>25%), pregnancy is still NOT advised in women with PHT.
- Women with PHT who have an unplanned pregnancy are advised to terminate the pregnancy unless the fetus can be delivered
- Women who wish to continue the pregnancy despite thorough counselling should be managed in a high risk dedicated centre with expertise in PHT in pregnancy.

Aetiology

PHT is characterized by luminal obliteration of the small pulmonary arterioles due to vascular remodeling. It is divided into:
- pulmonary arterial HT
- pulmonary HT with left heart disease
- pulmonary HT associated with lung disease or hypoxaemia
- pulmonary HT secondary to chronic thromboembolic disease
- miscellaneous, e.g. sarcoid, scleroderma.

Definition

On cardiac catheter:
- mean PA pressure >25 mmHg at rest or 30 mmHg on exercise
- PCW pressure must be <15 mmHg
- pulmonary vascular resistance >240 dynes/s/cm^2.

Presentation

- SOB in absence of overt cardiac or pulmonary disease.
- Can also present with:
  - chest pain
  - syncope
  - fatigue
  - weakness
  - Abdo distension.

Physical signs

- RV heave.
- Loud P2.
- Pansystolic murmur of TR.
- Diastolic murmur of PR.
- RV 3rd HS.

If advanced and RV failing, may also have:
- cold extremities
- raised JVP
- hepatomegaly
- peripheral oedema.

Diagnosis
- ECG & CXR abnormal in 90% patients with PHT.
  - ECG—RVH and strain, RA dilatation.
- Echo.
  - Most useful non-invasive test.
- Lung function test.
  - To detect coincidental lung disease.
- CTPA—to diagnose or exclude thromboembolic disease.
- Cardiac catheterization to measure pressures.

Treatment
ADVISE AGAINST CONTINUING THE PREGNANCY

If patient elects to continue:
- anticoagulation
  - whilst VTE disease is a cause of PHT, patients with PHT have a high incidence of vascular thrombotic lesions
- oxygen
  - reduces PVR in both hypoxic and non-hypoxic patients
- disease targeted therapies
  - prostanoids—many different formulations for acute and chronic use
  - calcium channel blockers—beneficial in patients with positive vasoreactivity test (<10% patients). Only half that respond acutely will have long-term benefit
  - phosphodiesterase inhibitors (PD 5) inhibitors, e.g. sildenafil
  - endothelin antagonists, e.g. Bosentan. This class of drugs is known to cause birth defects in animals but if their use has resulted in improvement or normalization of pulmonary pressures prior to pregnancy, then the benefit to the mother of continuing them in pregnancy probably outweighs any theoritical risk to the fetus
- monitor right heart during pregnancy with echo
- aim to deliver by 36–37th week at latest.

Delivery
- Full high risk delivery team required.
- Be prepared for early delivery.
- Consider use of inhaled nitric oxide during delivery.
- Careful cardiac obstetric anaesthesia, i.e. epidural and reduced fluids.
- No prolonged valsalva manouevre.
- PA catheter usually not required.
- Many will need caesarean section due to combination of fetal prematurity and maternal condition.
- Consider use of B Lynch suture prophylactically to prevent post partum haemorrhage (PPH). It reduces the need for uterotonics some of which (syntocinon) cause vasodilation.
- Women will need early anticoagulation post-natally but tolerate blood loss poorly, hence the need for flexibility depending on the relative risks of thrombosis and bleeding.
- Monitor post-natally on ITU/high dependency area.
- Women with PHT are most at risk up to 72 hours following delivery.

Conclusion

- PHT remains a complex disease with a high maternal mortality.
- Pregnancy is contraindicated in these women.
- Women who decline advice to avoid pregnancy should be supported by a multidisciplinary team with expertise in the management of pulmonary hypertension in pregnancy.

Aortic pathology

Coarctation of the aorta

- Stenosis of the descending aorta, typically distal to the origin of the left subclavian artery (uncomplicated, 'adult type').
- It accounts for 5–8% of congenital heart disease.
- 'Infantile' type coarctation includes hypoplastic aortic arch and coarctation can occur anywhere along the arch, involving a variety of head-and-neck vessels.
- Severity of stenosis predicts presence and extent of collaterals.
- Frequently (up to 85%) associated with bicuspid aortic valve.
- Aortopathy is present and may cause ascending aortic dilatation.

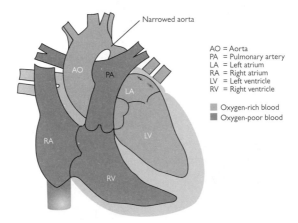

Narrowed aorta

AO = Aorta
PA = Pulmonary artery
LA = Left atrium
RA = Right atrium
LV = Left ventricle
RV = Right ventricle

■ Oxygen-rich blood
■ Oxygen-poor blood

Fig. 12.1 Coarcation of the aorta.

Presentation
- Murmur
  - Continuous and/or late systolic murmur heard best over the thoracic spine.
  - Associated with abnormal pulses—radio-femoral delay, i.e. pulses distal to the obstruction are diminished.
- Hypertension.

Complications of coarctation
- Uncontrolled hypertension—may be diagnosed for the first time in pregnancy.
- Left ventricular hypertrophy.
- Stroke.
- Aortic dissection, especially during pregnancy or the puerperium and if ascending aorta is dilated.
- LV decompensation if coarctation is tight.

Management
Relief of coarctation
- Surgical procedure including:
  - end-to-end anastomosis (risk of restenosis)
  - patch repair (risk of aneurysm formation at the repair site)
  - subclavian flap repair (aneurysm formation is a risk).
- Angioplasty +/− stent implantation.

Management of hypertension
- Beta-blockers are often used due to their ability to reduce sheer stress along aorta.

Complications post coarctation repair
Hypertension
- Common even after successful repair.
- As with other patients who have hypertension, patients are at risk of premature coronary disease, heart failure and rupture of aneurysms (aortic or cerebral).

Recoarctation
- Can occur between 3–40% of cases.
- Women with previous surgical repair should have regular imaging follow-up, especially prior to embarking on pregnancy.
- Echo can identify turbulant flow and gradients across a recoarctation however CT or MRI are the imaging modalities of choice.
- Restenosis or aneurysm formation should be treated before conception.

Aneurysm of the ascending aorta (See Figure 12.2)
- Occur in 5–9% of postoperative patients.
- The risk of dissection or aneurysm rupture is higher during pregnancy, related to increased haemodynamic burden and the effects of progesterone on connective tissue.
- Rupture can be life threatening.

Infective endocarditis
- See Chapter 6.

Aneurysms of the circle of Willis
- Berry aneurysms of the circle of Willis or other vessels occurs in 10%.

Implications for pregnancy
- Hypertension exacerbated in pregnancy:
  - manage as discussed in Chapter 15 but beta-blockers should be used to protect the aorta even in the 1st trimester
- Stress of labour may need to be reduced with:
  - early epidural
  - assisted second stage (ventouse or forceps).
- Recurrence risk of coarctation in child
  - 2% if 1 sibling affected, 6% if 2 are affected.

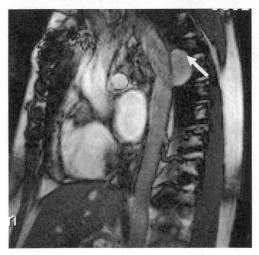

Fig. 12.2 This MRI is of a 32 yr old female who was 22 weeks' pregnant. It demonstrates a pseudoaneurysm of the aorta at the site of a previous coarctation repair (marked).

Marfan syndrome

- Autosomal dominant condition of connective tissue. Involves:
  - cardiovascular
  - skeletal
  - ocular abnormalities
  - less common – pulmonary, skin and CNS abnormalities.
- Occurs in 1 in 3,000–5,000 people.
- Secondary to an abnormality of the fibrillin 1 gene (FBN 1).

Diagnosis

- Occurrence of major manifestations in two different categories and involvement of a third category.
- See Table 12.1.

Complications

- Aortic dissection:
  - risk increased with dilating aorta; however patients with normal sized aorta can also dissect.

Management to reduce risk of aortic dissection

- Beta blockers have been shown to slow rate of aortic dilatation and reduce the risk of dissection.
- Avoidance of heavy exertion, e.g. isometric exertion and contact sports.
- Surgical intervention in the dilating aorta:
  - pregnancy should be avoided in women with an aorta >45mm until surgical repair has been carried out.

Implications for pregnancy

- Increased risk of aortic dissection during pregnancy and up to 6 months post-partum.
- There is a 50% chance the baby will be affected.
- Stress of labour may need to be reduced with:
  - early epidural
  - assisted second stage.
- It is important to know if a woman has dural ectasia as this means regional analgesia/anaesthesia is contraindicated.

Table 12.1 Diagnostic criteria for Marfan syndrome[a]

Criterion	Major	Minor
Family history	Independent diagnosis in parent, child, sibling	None
Genetics	Mutation of *FBN1*	None
Cardiovascular	Aortic root dilatation	Mitral valve prolapse
	Dissection of ascending aorta	Calcification of the mitral valve (<40 years)
		Dilatation of pulmonary artery
		Dilatation or dissection of descending aorta
Ocular	Ectopia lentis	(Two needed): flat cornea
		myopia
		elongated globe
Skeletal	(Four needed):pectus excavatum needing operation	(Two major, or one major and two minor signs): moderate pectus excavatum
	pectus carinatum	high, narrowly arched palate
	pes planus	typical facies
	wrist *and* thumb sign	joint hypermobility
	scoliosis>20° or spondylolisthesis	
	arm span: height ratio>1.05	
	protrusio acetabulae (X-ray, MRI)	
	diminished extension elbows(<170°)	
Pulmonary		Spontaneous pneumothorax
		Apical bulla
Skin		Unexplained stretch marks (striae)
		Recurrent or incisional herniae
Central nervous system	Lumbosacral dural ectasia (CT or MRI)	

[a]Requires the presence of major criteria in two of six separate systems and the involvement of a third system. If family history is felt to be positive, *at least* one family member needs to have met these criteria without the use of family history (two of five major systems positive pulse a third system). Reproduced from Gatzoulis, Webb and Daubeney (2010) *Diagnosis and Management of Adult Congenital Heart Disease* with permission from Elsevier.

Loeys-Dietz syndrome

- Autosomal dominant genetic syndrome with features similar to Marfans.
- Mutation in transforming growth factor.

Features

- Aortic and arterial aneurysms/dissection.
- Hypertelorism (widely spaced eyes).
- Cleft palate.

Less common features

- Scoliosis.
- Pectus excavatum.
- Long fingers and joint hypermobility.
- Club foot.
- Congenital heart defects including:
  - PDA
  - ASD
  - bicuspid aortic valve.
- Pale thin skin.
- Dural ectasia.

Management

Management of these women should be as for Marfans but as it is a recently discovered syndrome, data in pregnancy are lacking.

Ehlers-Danlos syndrome

A group of heritable connective tissue disorders characterized by:
- hypermobile joints
- hyperelasticity and fragility of the skin
- dilatation and rupture of major arteries.

10 recognised forms, however Type IV is the one which raises concern in pregnancy because of the risk of aortic dissection.

Type IV EDS
- Autosomal dominant condition.
- Affects type III collagen.
- Rare – affects 1 in 100,000 to 250,000 patients.

Diagnosis
- Typical facial features:
  - large eyes
  - small chin
  - thin nose and lips
  - lobeless ears.
- Small stature and slim build.
- Pale translucent skin prone to bruising.
- Generalized features of EDS include:
  - highly flexible fingers and toes
  - hypermobility of major joints therefore prone to dislocations
  - high narrow palate
  - flat feet
  - prone to bruising
  - abnormal wound healing and scar formation
  - muscle weakness
  - osteoarthritis occurs much earlier than normal population
  - skin hyperelasticity
  - dystonia
  - mitral valve prolapse
  - nerve compression disorders.
- Gene mutations in COL3A1.

Management
- Joint supports.
- Recommend woman carries a medicalert bracelet.
- Reduce risk of trauma.
- Try and avoid surgery unless necessary.

Implications for pregnancy
- Risk of aortic dissection is up to 25% and therefore a greater risk than the Marfan patient.
- Increased risk of premature rupture of membranes.
- Risk of uterine rupture.
- Platelet aggregation failure therefore increased risk of bleeding.
- Pelvic pain and instability.
- Spinal deformities may make siting of epidural difficult.
- 50% of offspring affected.

Cyanotic heart disease

Introduction

Cyanosis is caused by insufficient oxygen content of systemic arterial blood. This may be due to:
- lack of oxygenation through the lungs
- or by mixing of adequately oxygenated arterial blood with venous blood through a right-to-left shunt:
  - usually happens when there is shunt reversal occurs, i.e. when pressures in the pulmonary circulation rise above systemic pressures and a previous left-to-right shunt becomes a right-to-left shunt (or bi-directional shunt). This is known as Eisenmenger syndrome
  - the shunt can be at any level and can be either within the heart, e.g. ASD, VSD, between the great vessels, e.g. PDA or extracardiac, i.e. intrapulmonary AV malformations.

General principles

With increasing cyanosis, the chance of carrying a fetus to term reduces dramatically from 92% for a woman with resting O_2 saturations above 90% to 12% if resting saturations are below 85%.

Problems encountered in pregnancy

There are certain situations which increase either the level of cyanosis or its clinical manifestations and thus should be avoided particularly in pregnant women:
1. Iron deficiency.
2. Systemic vasodilators – increase right to left shunting.
3. Dehydration can lead to worsening renal impairment.
4. Tachyarrhythmias.
5. Cerebral abscesses – women are more prone to infection in pregnancy and cyanotic patients are already prone to cerebral abscesses due to shunts.

Table 13.1 Non-cardiac manifestations of cyanosis

Blood & vessels	Erythrocytosis secondary to hypoxia
	Thrombocytopenia
	Coagulopathy; haemorrhage or thrombosis
	Iron deficiency secondary to over-venesection or menorrhagia
	Atherosclerotic coronary disease - rare
Neurological	CVA secondary to paradoxical embolism
	Cerebral abscess
Renal	Renal impairment due to glomerular proteinuria, mesangial matrix thickening, capillary and hilar arteriole dilatation
	Risk of iatrogenic renal failure if dehydrated or renal toxic medication
Skin & bones	Acne
	Gout
	Digital clubbing
	Hypertrophic osteoarthropathy
Gastro-intestinal	Gallstones

*Adapted from Thorne & Clift, 2009 *Oxford Handbook of Adult Congenital Heart Disease.* Oxford University Press.

Maternal risk in cyanotic heart disease

Cyanotic heart disease without PHT

Maternal risk during pregnancy largely depends on whether or not pulmonary hypertension (Eisenmenger syndrome in the context of congenital heart disease) is present or not.

In the absence of pulmonary hypertension, maternal risk is determined by the following factors:

- ventricular function:
  - if ventricular function (systemic or sub-pulmonary) is already impaired pre-pregnancy, the additional volume load and work related to the physiological changes of pregnancy may precipitate heart failure.
- thromboembolism:
  - cyanotic patients with congenital heart disease shunt right-to-left, which means they are at risk of paradoxical embolism. This risk increases during pregnancy because of the physiological hypercoagulability.
- deranged coagulation:
  - impaired platelet function and a consumptive coagulopathy may be associated with cyanotic heart disease and right-to-left shunting.
- increase in right-to-left shunt during pregnancy:
  - a pregnancy related fall in systemic vascular resistance increases right-to-left shunting, causing lower systemic oxygen saturations and cyanosis. Symptomatically, the woman may feel more breathless. Systemic vasodilators can exacerbate this.

Cyanotic heart disease with PHT

- In the presence of pulmonary hypertension (Eisenmenger syndrome or any other cause of PHT), maternal risk increases dramatically
- The reported risk of death during pregnancy for a woman with pulmonary hypertension is between 25 and 40%, with a slight fall in the last decade, perhaps due to advanced therapies
- Death occurs during pregnancy or in the post-partum period (usually within the first month of delivery) and may occur suddenly or through a downward spiral of refractory hypoxia.

The risk of pregnancy remains extremely high and such women should be advised against pregnancy. If pregnancy occurs, therapeutic termination should be offered, which in itself carries significant mortality.

If the woman elects to continue the pregnancy, a multidisciplinary approach is necessary to facilitate the best possible outcome.

Management of a pregnant woman with PHT is discussed in Chapter 10.

Specific cyanotic lesions

Tetralogy of Fallot (ToF) (Figures 13.1 and 2)
'Classic' tetralogy includes ventricular septal defect with the aorta overriding the VSD, subpulmonary stenosis and secondary right ventricular hypertrophy:
- commonest cyanotic lesion, 1:3600 live births
- wide range of morphological variation (minimal pulmonary stenosis to pulmonary atresia, small VSD with minimal 'override' to double outlet left ventricle)
- often associated with ASD, persistent left sided SVC, right sided aortic arch, aortopulmonary collaterals.

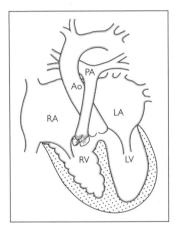

Fig. 13.1 Schematic representation of unoperated tetralogy of Fallot. * deviation of outlet septum, Ao aorta; LA left atrium; LV left ventricle; PA pulmonary artery; RA right atrium; RV right ventricle.
Reproduced with permission from Thorne S, Clift P (2009) *Adult Congenital Heart Disease.* Oxford University Press.

NB: Di George syndrome (chromosome 22q11 deletion) has similar cardiac defects in association with facial abnormalities (cleft palate and hair lip) and learning difficulties. There is a high risk of recurrence in the off-spring therefore genetic counselling should be offered in such cases.

Most patients undergoing a pregnancy will have had some form of surgical repair (see below) however, ToF may present during pregnancy if women survive undiagnosed to adulthood (~2%). Typical presentations of uncorrected ToF during pregnancy include:
- atrial or ventricular arrhythmia
- increasing cyanosis due to fall in SVR

- ventricular failure–Increase in plasma volume during pregnancy may precipitate ventricular failure in already volume loaded ventricle, especially if aortic regurgitation is present
- aortic dilatation (less risk of dissection than in the patient with Marfan syndrome).

Pregnancy in unoperated patients is high risk with fetal loss as high as 30% and maternal mortality between 4 and 15%. The decrease in peripheral resistance may increase right to left shunt rendering the women more cyanotic.

Surgical treatment patient may have previously had:
- Shunt palliation (mostly historical):
  - the Blalock-Taussig or BT shunt (left or right) increases pulmonary blood flow by connecting subclavian or innominate arteries to the pulmonary artery thus bypassing the RV and its obstruction
  - patients remain cyanotic as the BT shunt creates a further systemic-pulmonary shunt
  - the historical Brock procedure refers to an RV infundibular resection to relieve RV outflow tract obstruction and increase pulmonary blood flow, decreasing the right-to-left shunt.
- Radical repair:
  - procedure of choice; involves patch closure of the VSD, resection of pulmonary infundibular stenosis and often a transannular patch to increase the size of the pulmonary annulus.

Typical complications
- Pulmonary regurgitation of varying degrees (if transannular patch used).
  - Usually well tolerated in pregnancy if RV function is preserved.
- Arrhythmia:
  - atrial or ventricular – this may be precipitated by pregnancy related increase in sympathetic tone or volume loading.
- Residual RV outflow tract obstruction.
  - Results in the inability to increase cardiac output and to cope with the haemodynamic stress of pregnancy.
  - May precipitate RV failure.
- Complete heart block:
  - may develop late following surgical repair and may require treatment during pregnancy.
- Sudden death:
  - likely arrhythmogenic in origin, therefore theoretically a higher risk during pregnancy, although limited data exist on this topic.

If a woman has a good surgical repair with stable haemodynamics, her risk of a pregnancy is low, approaching that of the general population. The risk increases in women with significant residual RVOT obstruction, severe PR with or without TR and RV dysfunction. Maternal deaths in women with surgically corrected ToF have mostly been related to impaired RV function.

All women with ToF should have pre-pregnancy assessment and counselling, genetic counseling with exclusion of 22q11 deletion and fetal echo during pregnancy.

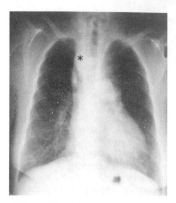

Fig. 13.2 Tetralogy of Fallot with R-sided aortic arch. Chest radiograph of a 24-year-old ♀ with repaired tetralogy of Fallot and a R-sided aortic arch (*). This anomaly is present in ~16% of patients with tetralogy of Fallot and is associated with chromosome 22q11 microdeletions.
Reproduced with permission from Thorne S, Clift P (2009) *Adult Congenital Heart Disease*. Oxford University Press.

Ebstein's anomaly

Definition: Apical displacement of the often structurally abnormal tricuspid valve. Results in large right atrium and small right ventricle, often with restrictive physiology.

• Rare: 1:20,000 live births.
• Associated with maternal lithium ingestion in the first trimester
• Commonly associated with ASD or PFO as well as Wolff-Parkinson-White syndrome (25%).

Patients may present in pregnancy if previously undiagnosed, typically with:

• increasing cyanosis:
  • restrictive RV physiology, septal defect and fall in SVR during pregnancy.
• arrhythmia:
  • increased propensity to arrhythmia during pregnancy combined with volume loading (on top of an already large right atrium)
• venous congestion:
  • symptoms of right heart failure even if RV systolic function preserved), depending on the degree of tricuspid regurgitation
• paradoxical embolism:
  • if shunt is present
• infective endocarditis.

Overall pregnancy is well tolerated in Ebstein's providing there is no significant cyanosis, arrhythmia, and or haemodynamic compromise.

Fetal loss is increased in women with cyanosis and overall, women have lower birth weight babies than the general population.

Univentricular hearts (see Figure 13.3a and b)

Refers to a variety of very complex congenital cardiac malformations, where one dominant ventricle supports both the systemic and pulmonary circulations. Common lesions include:

- tricuspid atresia
- pulmonary atresia with intact ventricular septum and small RV
- hypoplastic left heart syndrome
- double inlet LV, often with transpositon of the great arteries and pulmonary stenosis
- complex AVSDs with left or right atrial isomerism.

Patients typically present as neonates and few survive to childhood without surgery. All have in common that correction to a biventricular circulation is not possible. Surgery is generally palliative and usually results in a form of Fontan circulation if surgery is possible. If left unoperated, the outcome is poor.

The Fontan circulation (see Figure 13.4)

Definition: Systemic venous blood is diverted into the lung bypassing the right or subpulmonary ventricle to separate lung and systemic circulations:

- Venous return to the lungs is passive (through negative intrathoracic pressure and 'suction' from the systemic ventricle) in the absence of a right or subpulmonary ventricle.
- This is a palliative operation for single ventricle physiology (see above).

Many variations of the Fontan operation exist:

- classic or AP-Fontan:
  - connects right atrium to pulmonary artery.
- extracardiac Fontan:
  - a conduit connects inferior vena cava directly to the pulmonary artery
- RA-RV Fontan (Bjoerk modification):
  - used if a small right ventricle is present.
    - Blood is directed from RA to RV to the lungs.
- total cavo-pulmonary connection (TCPC-Fontan):
  - inferior vena cava connects directly to the right pulmonary artery, the superior vena cava connects to right and/or left pulmonary artery
  - often a small fenestration is left, creating a small right-to-left shunt, to reduce venous pressure and increase cardiac output
  - the TCPC Fontan is the operation of choice since the early 1990s and is considered least 'thrombogenic'.

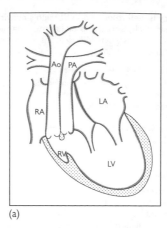

(a)

Fig. 13.3a Schematic representation of univentricular heart; a double inlet LV with VA discordance. Ao aorta; LA left atrium; LV left ventricle; PA pulmonary artery; RA right atrium; RV right ventricle.
Reproduced with permission from Thorne S, Clift P (2009). *Adult Congenital Heart Disease*. Oxford University Press.

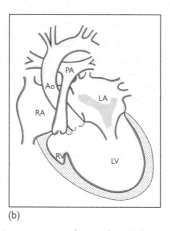

(b)

Fig. 13.3b Schematic representation of tricuspid atresia. Ao aorta; LA left atrium; LV left ventricle; PA pulmonary artery; RA right atrium; RV right ventricle.
Reproduced with permission from Throne S, Clift P (2009). *Adult Congenital Heart Disease*. Oxford University Press.

Complications post Fontan procedure
- Right atrial dilatation.
- Atrial arrhythmias (very common and may be life-threatening as poorly tolerated).
- Sinus node dysfunction.
- Systemic AV valve regurgitation.
- Sluggish blood flow within the venous system with risk of thrombus formation.
- High venous pressures.
- Obstruction of Fontan or pulmonary venous pathway obstruction.
- Protein losing enteropathy in ~10%.
- Systemic ventricular failure.
- Cyanosis (due to collateral formation or through iatrogenic fenestration).
- Infective endocarditis.

In the biggest series of pregnancy in women with Fontan circulation there were no deaths however there was significant maternal morbidity and fetal mortality. Almost half of women suffered significant atrial arrhythmias whilst a decline in NYHA class was common. Overt heart failure was seen in just fewer than 10% and interestingly, post partum, the majority of women recover their functional status to baseline. There is a high spontaneous miscarriage rate (up to 50%) which may be a reflection of the fact these women are usually fully anticoagulated. However, if the fetus survives beyond the first trimester, outcome is good.

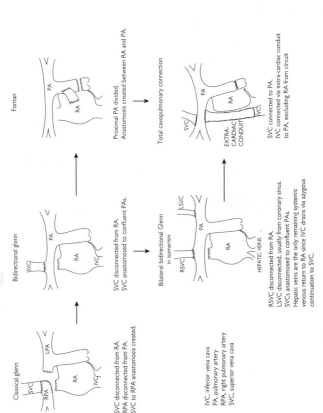

Fig. 13.4 Evolution of Fontan and total cavopulmonary connection.

Acyanotic congenital heart disease

Introduction

Acyanotic patients are 'pink'. Conditions without cyanosis may have no communication between systemic and pulmonary circulation (i.e. no shunt), or may have a left-to-right shunt.

Specific lesions

- Septal defects (PFO, ASD, AVSD, VSD).
- Transposition of the great arteries (TGA).
- Pulmonary atresia with ventricular septal defect (VSD).

Patent foramen ovale (PFO)

- A remnant of the fetal circulation, present in 10–20% of the population.
- Rarely causes problems, unless paradoxical embolism occurs or the left-to-right shunt is large (exceedingly rare).
- Percutaneous closure may be indicated, but this is almost never required during pregnancy.
- Thromboprophylaxis may be necessary in pregnant patients with a previous history of paradoxical embolism.

Atrial septal defect (ASD)

- Commonest congenital abnormality (~10% of all congenital lesions).
- Frequently present in adulthood if no associated lesions present.
- Ostium secundum defects make up ~75% of ASD's, often occur in isolation.
- Ostium primum defects often have comcomitant mitral valve abnormalities (then referred to as AVSDs).
- Sinus venosus defects are rarest and commonly associated with anomalous pulmonary venous drainage.

Left-to-right shunt at atrial level.

- If large results in volume overload of the right heart (atrium and ventricle).
- Closure (surgical or percutaneous, depending on anatomy and associated malformations) is recommended if shunt ratio is >1.5:1, or if there are signs of right heart volume/pressure overload.
- This should be done outside pregnancy.

Complications of uncorrected ASDs

- Right heart dilatation and rise in right heart pressure, leading to shunt reversal (Eisenmenger syndrome).
- Paradoxical embolism.
- Atrial arrhythmia, often unmasked in pregnancy (may also require anticoagulation).
- Failure of an already volume loaded and dilated RV, precipitated by plasma volume expansion during pregnancy.
- Eisenmenger syndrome (i.e. shunt reversal, see Chapter 12).

The only contraindication to pregnancy in women with ASDs, operated or not, is persisting pulmonary hypertension. Otherwise, this is a low risk lesion though women do need assessing by a cardiologist as to whether they require anticoagulation/aspirin through pregnancy and every effort should be taken to avoid thrombosis. Lesions which are particularly susceptible are those associated with very large atria size, women at high risk of thrombosis, e.g. prolonged bed rest or women with previous arrhythmia.

Closed ASDs do not require any specific management during pregnancy and can be treated as normal unless there is persisting pulmonary hypertension.

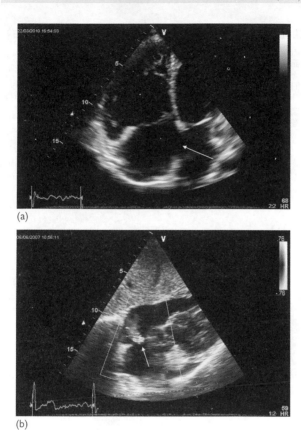

Fig. 14.1 (a) Here on this apical 4 chamber view, the defect in the atrial septum can clearly be seen (marked), along with a dilated right side of the heart due to increased flow across the defect. (b) In this smaller ASD, flow is seen across the septum on colour flow in this subcostal view.

Atrio-ventricular septal defects (AVSDs)

- Refers to a variety of lesions of the atrial septum combined with anomalies of the mitral and/or tricuspid valves and/or the ventricular septum.
- There is an association with Trisomy 21 (Down's syndrome).
- Complications are largely dependent on the physiology associated with the morphological abnormality and include left-to-right shunting, volume overload, arrhythmia and AV valvular regurgitation.

Ventricular septal defects (VSD)

Can occur in isolation or as part of complex congenital lesions such as Tetralogy of Fallot:

- if small, they are well tolerated in pregnancy
- if large closure is indicated, ideally prior to pregnancy.

General complications (not specific to pregnancy)

- LV volume overload with long-standing left-to-right shunt at ventricular level.
- LV failure – if LV systolic function is poor may require thromboprophylaxis during pregnancy.
- Arrhythmia.
- There are case reports of heart failure occurring in women with large VSDs so these women should have specialist follow up.

Corrected VSDs. Like ASDs, can be treated as normal during pregnancy.

- Patients who have had a VSD closed and have normal PA pressures have no increase risk with pregnancy however women with PHT should be advised against pregnancy (see Chapter 11).

The recurrence risk of congenital HD in offspring of women with VSD is approximately 3%.

Complete transposition of the great arteries (TGA)

- Also known as:
  - D-TGA (Fig. 14.2).
  - Atrio-ventricular concordance.
  - Ventriculo-arterial discordance.
- Lesion entails:
  - systemic veins (IVC and SVC) drain into RA, RV, then aorta
  - pulmonary venous return is to LA, LV, then PA, i.e. complete separation of systemic and pulmonary circulations, hence obligate shunt (otherwise non-compatible with life).

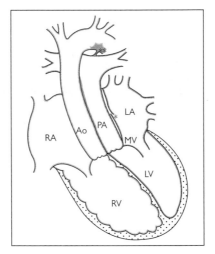

Fig. 14.2 Schematic representation of complete TGA (ventriculoarterial discordance). Ao aorta; LV left ventricle; PA pulmonary artery; MV mitral valve; RA right atrium; RV right ventricle; TV tricuspid valve. ** patient foramen ovale. * patient arterial duct. Reproduced with permission from Thorne S and Clift P (2009). *Adult Congenital Heart Disease*. Oxford University Press.

Surgical treatment

Arterial switch
- Procedure of choice for correction of complete TGA.
- Aorta and pulmonary artery are switched over and re-anastomosed to achieve ventriculo-arterial concordance.
- The coronaries need to be re-implanted into the neo-aorta (i.e. the previous pulmonary artery).

Complications
- Generally, typical complications arise from the anastomosis sites.
- The operation is performed within the first months of life, hence supra-aortic, supra-pulmonary and ostial coronary stenoses may occur.
- These may be unmasked through the haemodynamic requirements of pregnancy and can present as breathlessness or angina.

Atrial switch operations/interatrial repair (Mustard and Senning)
- Both rarely performed nowadays as patients are left with a systemic RV.
- However, many patients who were operated on before the 1980's may still present in pregnancy.
  - Mustard: Baffle from synthetic material or pericardium directs systemic venous return into the LV and into the lungs.
  - Senning: Baffle from native atrial tissue directs systemic venous return into LV and then the lungs.

Complications
- Atrial arrhythmias, typically flutter, often poorly tolerated and life-threatening if 1:1 conducted.
- Arrhythmogenicity of pregnancy and associated plasma expansion may precipitate this and cause decompensation.
- Urgent DC cardioversion and restoration of sinus rhythm may be life-saving.

Overall, in patients with good or only mildly impaired ventricular function and no previous arrhythmias, maternal risk from pregnancy is low.

There is a small risk of deterioration of ventricular function particularly in those with atrial switch repairs and in those women in NYHA 2 or higher.

Patients with impaired LV function and previous arrhythmias are at a higher risk of complications (see p. 276 Toronto risk score Siu data) and should be counselled appropriately.

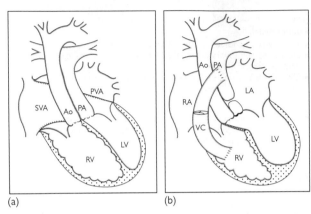

(a)   (b)

Fig. 14.3 Surgical approaches to complete TGA. a) Schematic representation of interatrial repair (Senning or Mustard operation). b) Schematic representation of Rastelli operation. Ao aorta; LA Left atrium; LV left ventricle; PA pulmonary artery; RA right atrium; RV right ventricle; VC valved conduit; PVA pulmonary venous atrium; SVA systemic venous atrium. Reproduced with permission from Thorne S and Clift P (2009). *Adult Congenital Heart Disease.* Oxford University Press.

Congenitally corrected TGA

Also known as L-TGA or ccTGA (see Fig.14.4)
- Discordance at atrio-ventricular level as well as ventriculo-arterial level, i.e. systemic venous blood returns to LA, then LV, then PA
- Pulmonary venous returns to RA, RV, then aorta, i.e. patients have a systemic RV.

Patients may present in adulthood, sometimes for the first time during pregnancy. A typical presentation in pregnancy may include:
- systemic RV failure precipitated by increased plasma volume and cardiac output
- pulmonary oedema—Low colloid osmotic pressure, potentially combined with systemic RV volume overload secondary to tricuspid valve regurgitation, may precipitate pulmonary oedema
- arrhythmia—Atrial or ventricular, depending on size and function of systemic atrium and ventricle, exacerbated or precipitated by pregnancy, and sometimes poorly tolerated.

Surgical repair

The double switch operation is a corrective anatomical repair (restoration of atrio-ventricular and ventriculo-arterial concordance).

Usually done early in life and rarely possible if the condition is only diagnosed in adulthood.

Review of the larger series of pregnancy in patients with CCTGA is encouraging. Maternal mortality is low and there were live births in 60-80% of pregnancies.

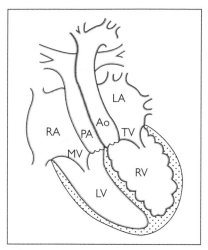

Fig. 14.4 Schematic represention of ccTGA (atrioventricular and ventriculoarterial discordance). Ao aorta; LA left atrium; LV left ventricle; PA pulmonary artery; RA right atrium; RV right ventricle; VC valved conduit; PVA pulmonary venous atrium; SVA syatemic venous atrium. Reproduced with permission from Thorne S and Clift P (2009). *Adult Congenital Heart Disease*. Oxford University Press.

Pulmonary atresia

- Blind-ending right ventricular outflow tract, only compatible with life if a shunt is present, typically a VSD but includes:
  - MAPCAs (major aortopulmonary collateral arteries – arise from descending aorta or its branches or bronchial arteries, connecting to pulmonary arteries)
  - multiple small collaterals from bronchial to pulmonary arteries.
- Depending on the anatomical variation, complete or partial repair may or may not be possible.
- Complications are similar to those seen in ToF and arise from increase in PVR and increasing cyanosis, particularly with fall in SVR during pregnancy, and from RV failure.

Hypertension

Definitions

Hypertension: consecutive blood pressure (BP) readings of $\geq$ 140/90 on more than one occasion at least 4 hours apart.

Incidence

- Hypertensive disorders are the commonest medical complications in pregnancy, affecting 10–15% of pregnant women.
- 3–5% of pregnant women develop pre-eclampsia which can result in serious maternal morbidity and mortality.
- Pre-eclampsia is the second commonest cause of direct maternal deaths in the UK.
- 20% of women with chronic hypertension develop superimposed pre-eclampsia.

Chronic/pre-existing hypertension:
Hypertension occurring pre-pregnancy or before 20 weeks' gestation.

Pregnancy-induced hypertension (PIH)/gestational hypertension
New-onset hypertension occurring $\geq$ 20 weeks' gestation.

Pre-eclampsia (PET)
New-onset hypertension occurring $\geq$ 20 weeks' gestation with significant proteinuria of $\geq$ 0.3g/24 hour.

Measurement of blood pressure in pregnant women

- Seated upright with arm supported at level of right atrium.
- Rested for 5 minutes before measurement.
- Use correct sized cuff: large cuff if arm circumference > 32 cm.
- Take diastolic pressure reading as when sounds disappear, i.e. Korotkoff phase V.

Treatment of hypertension in pregnancy

Aims of antihypertensive treatment

- To prevent maternal complications of cerebral haemorrhage from severe hypertension by keeping BP < 160/110 mmHg. The recent increase in maternal deaths in pre-eclampsia/eclampsia from intracranial haemorrhage are associated with a failure to control systolic BP to < 160 mmHg.
- To prevent acute hypertensive episodes which can result in early delivery. Does not influence progression of pre-eclampsia.
- To maintain adequate utero-placental perfusion and prevent fetal growth restriction by not lowering BP excessively or too rapidly.

When to prescribe antihypertensive in pregnancy

- Treat at any gestation if blood pressure is consistently >150/100 mmHg.
- Maintain the blood pressure at 130–150/80-100 mmHg, not lower.

Antihypertensive agents see Table 15.1

- First line. Commonly used agents are methyldopa, nifedipine (slow release) and labetolol. There are no evidence that one agent is better than another, although labetolol is contraindicated in women with asthma. Drugs can be used in combination. Methyldopa-induced hepatitis rare.
- Second line. Other oral drugs which can be used are amlodipine, doxazocin and hydralazine.
- Drugs not recommended in pregnancy are:
  - angiotensin enzyme (ACE) inhibitors and angiotensin receptor blockers (ARBs): 1st trimester teratogenic; 2nd and 3rd trimesters cause renal tubular dysplasia, anuria, oligohydramnios, hypocalvaria, dysmorphic features, and fetal growth restriction (FGR). Fetal renal failure and intrauterine death can occur.
  - diuretics: reduce intravascular volume which is already constricted in pre-eclampsia. Furosemide is used in pre-eclampsia with pulmonary oedema.
  - atenolol: associated with FGR particularly if used in high doses in the 1st trimester.

Table 15.1 Oral anti hypertensives used in pregnancy

Drug	Action	Dose	Main side effects	Contraindications
Methyldopa	Centrally acting	250 mg tds to 1 g tds (or 750 mg qds)	Sedation	Depression
Nifedipine slow release	Calcium channel blocker	10 mg bd to 40 mg bd	Headaches, leg oedema, flushing, palpitations	Aortic stenosis
Labetolol	α and β blocker	100 mg tds to 800 mg tds	Bronchospasm, bradycardia	Asthma Phaeochromocytoma
Amlodipine	Calcium channel blocker	5mg od to 10 mg od	Leg oedema	Aortic stenosis
Doxazocin	α-blocker	1 mg od to 8 mg bd	Postural hypotension	
Hydralazine	Vasodilator	25 mg bd to 50 mg bd	Headaches, flushing, tachycardia, palpitations	HR > 120 bpm

Post-partum management of hypertension

Do not use:
- Methyldopa – causes depression.

Use any of the following (in combination if necessary):
- atenolol
- nifedipine slow release
- enalapril – most data for this older ACE inhibitor in breast feeding
- amlodipine.

- β-blockers, calcium channel antagonists, and ACE inhibitors are safe in breastfeeding.
- Change labetolol to atenolol post-partum (better compliance with *od* drug).
- Maintain blood pressure control at ≤150/100 mmHg.

Gestational hypertension and pre-eclampsia:
- BP falls to normal range in a few weeks
- intracerebral bleeds and eclampsia are rare after the 3rd post-partum day
- if still hypertensive >6 weeks post-partum, exclude secondary causes (e.g. hyperaldosteronism and phaeochromocytoma)
- avoid diuretics for 6 weeks post-partum in women with pre-eclampsia (unless pulmonary oedema).

Chronic hypertension:
- Recommence pre-pregnancy treatment or start on *od* drugs, e.g. enalapril, amlodipine.

Pre-eclampsia

Multisystem disorder in pregnancy of unknown aetiology characterized by the presence of hypertension and proteinuria. It can become rapidly progressive and affects both the mother and fetus.

Pathology

Poor placentation with inadequate trophoblastic invasion and remodelling of the spiral arteries. Placental ischaemia causes a harmful maternal inflammatory response with oxidative stress which results in widespread endothelial dysfunction. This causes a maternal syndrome and fetal syndrome.

Risk factors

- Ethnicity (afrocaribbean).
- First pregnancy.
- Age > 35.
- ≥10 years since last baby.
- Obesity, BMI > 35.
- Family history pre-eclampsia in mother/sister.
- Previous pre-eclampsia.
- Multiple pregnancies.
- Pre-existing medical conditions:
  - chronic hypertension
  - chronic renal disease
  - diabetes mellitus
  - systemic lupus erythematosus
  - antiphospholipid syndrome.

Clinical symptoms

(May be absent even in severe disease):
- progressive swelling: limbs and face
- headaches
- visual disturbance particularly blurred vision
- epigastric or right upper quadrant pain
- nausea or vomiting.

Clinical signs

- Hypertension (vasoconstriction).
- Proteinuria ≥ 1+ on dipstick (glomerular damage).
- Peripheral and facial oedema (extravasation of fluid though leaky capillaries).
- Hyperreflexia or clonus ('cerebral irritability').
- Epigastric or right upper quadrant tenderness.
- Confusion.
- Papilloedema.

Complications

Maternal syndrome
- Eclampsia (seizures: cerebral oedema).
- HELLP syndrome (haemolysis, elevated liver enzymes, low platelets).
- Hepatic subcapsular haematoma.
- Renal impairment.
- Pulmonary oedema.
- Disseminated intravascular coagulation.
- Retinal detachments (retinal oedema).
- Cortical blindness (cerebral occipital oedema).
- Placental abruption.

Fetal syndrome
- Fetal growth restriction.
- Stillbirth.
- Iatrogenic preterm delivery.
- Neonatal morbidity and mortality.

Investigations
- Pre-eclampsia blood tests (PET body) (and abnormalities that occur in pre-eclampsia):
  - U+E (raised creatinine i.e. >80μmol/L)
  - FBC (low platelets, raised haematocrit)
  - LFT (abnormal transaminases)
  - urate (raised)
  - clotting (if platelets < 100×10^9).
- 24 hour urine collection (≥ 0.3 g/d proteinuria: equivalent to a protein:creatinine ratio ≥ 30).
- MSU (to exclude UTI as a cause for proteinuria).
- Cardiotocograph (CTG) if gestation > 26 weeks.
- Fetal ultrasound scan: fetal growth, estimated fetal weight, amniotic fluid volume, umbilical artery Doppler flow velocity waveform.

Antenatal management
As an inpatient for intensive surveillance as pre-eclampsia is progressive:
- 4 hourly BP measurements
- treat with antihypertensives if BP consistently ≥ 150/100 mmHg
- alternate day PET bloods
- fetal surveillance: daily fetal CTG, serial growth scans.

Treatment of pre-eclampsia
- The only treatment for pre-eclampsia is delivery.
- Delivery at early gestations can result in significant neonatal morbidity and mortality (see Table 22.5, Chapter 22).
- The growth restricted fetus has poorer outcomes compared to babies delivered very preterm through spontaneous pre-term labour.

- Expectant management is employed up to 34 weeks' gestation if possible, beyond which the fetal lungs are mature. This is balanced against maternal deterioration.
- Fetal lung maturity is promoted by administration of betamethasone (2 doses of 12 mg 12–24 hours apart) between 24 to 34 weeks' gestation.
- At any gestation, the maternal condition takes priority over the fetus. This may require termination of a pregnancy with severe early-onset pre-eclampsia at < 24 weeks' gestation.

Management of hypertension antenatally in pre-eclampsia
See treatment of hypertension section, p.194.

Management of acute severe hypertension
Defined as a BP ≥ 160/110 mmHg:

- Check BP with a manual sphygmomanometer as automated readings underestimate the diastolic BP.
- Oral treatments with either nifedipine short acting 10 mg stat (not sublingual which causes abrupt hypotension and fetal distress), or labetolol 200 mg.
- Intravenous agents are used if the BP is not controlled with these oral agents, or patient is vomiting or nil by mouth: use labetolol or hydralazine (see Table 15.2). May need intravenous infusions.
- If the BP very difficult to control then may need invasive monitoring with an arterial line.
- PET bloods, clotting and group and save as delivery may be necessary.
- Strict hourly fluid balance to prevent pulmonary oedema: total fluid input 80 ml/h. Usually need urinary catheterization.
- Central venous pressure (CVP) line if oliguria or pulmonary oedema
- Fetal assessment with CTG.
- $MgSO_4$ if fulminating pre-eclampsia and/or delivery planned.
- Thromboprophylaxis if immediate delivery not planned and no coagulopathy, due to increased risks of thrombosis.

Table 15.2 Intravenous antihypertensive for the treatment of acute severe hypertension (BP ≥ 160/110 mmHg)

Drug	Dosage	Additions	Contraindications
Labetolol	20 mg, then 40 mg then 80 mg at 15 minutely intervals. Then start infusion of 20 mg/h to a max of 160 mg/h	-	Asthma phaeochromocytoma
Hydralazine	5 mg over 5 min. Max 3 doses at 15 minutely intervals. Then start infusion of 5 mg/h	Preload with 250 ml colloid before administration	HR > 120 bpm

Indications for delivery:
- Uncontrolled hypertension despite maximal antihypertensive treatment.
- Maternal symptoms (headaches, visual disturbances etc).
- HELLP syndrome.
- Renal impairment.
- Pulmonary oedema.
- Eclampsia.
- Coagulopathy.
- Fetal distress.

Management at delivery

Aim for a vaginal delivery. Induction of labour is often necessary. Caesarean section for obstetric indications or if urgent delivery is necessary for maternal or fetal reasons:
- 15 minutely BP readings until stable, then hourly
- PET bloods, clotting if pre-eclampsial platelets <100, group and save
- fluid restrict to 80 ml/h
- monitor fluid balance
- continuous fetal monitoring if in labour
- continue oral antihypertensive agents
- treat acute hypertension as above
- magnesium sulphate for prophylaxis against eclampsia if fulminating pre-eclampsia
- regional analgesia helps reduce blood pressure
- Third stage: use syntocinon, avoid ergometrine.

Postnatal management
- In moderate and severe pre-eclampsia, maintain fluid restriction for 12-24 hours post-partum.
- If on $MgSO_4$ for seizure prophylaxis, continue this for 24 hours post-partum.
- Consider thromboprophylaxis with LMWH.
- Maintain BP ≤150/100 mmHg with antihypertensives (see above).

Recurrence
10% if late onset pre-eclampsia. Higher if severe-early onset pre-eclampsia.

Prevention of pre-eclampsia in future pregnancies
- Low dose aspirin (75 mg od).
- Calcium (at least 1 g) in those with low calcium intake.

Future risk
- Pre-eclampsia is a predictor for future cardiovascular disease.
- Doubles future risk of hypertension, ischaemic heart disease, and stroke.
- Limit these risks by lifestyle modification and treatment of other identified risk factors.

Thrombo-embolic disease

Thrombophilias

- Inherited (15% of the Caucasian population) or acquired (antiphospholipid antibodies).
- Present in 50% of those with VTE in pregnancy.
- Most thrombogenic are antithrombin deficiency, homozygosity for Factor V Leiden (FVL) and G20210A prothrombin gene mutation and compound thrombophilias (see Table 16.2).
- Thrombotic risk in women with thrombophilia further ↑ if had a previous VTE or family history of VTE.
- Selective screening appropriate for women:
  - who develop VTE in pregnancy
  - with a personal history of VTE
  - with a family history of VTE.

Diagnosis of venous thrombo-embolism (VTE)

- Clinical assessment of VTE is not reliable for diagnosis. Many clinical features of DVT/PTE occur in normal pregnancy (e.g. leg oedema, dyspnoea, ECG abnormalities raised D-dimer)
- Obtain objective evidence of a VTE.

Effects of pregnancy on thrombophilia screen
- Protein S falls
- Activated protein C resistance (APCR) rises: test for Factor V Leiden by PCR (can be done in pregnancy)
- If extensive thrombus, antithrombin falls
- If patient has nephrotic syndrome or pre-eclampsia antithrombin falls
- If patient has liver disease, Protein S and Protein C fall.

Table 16.2 Thrombogenicity of the inherited thrombophilias

Inherited thrombophilia		Incidence of VTE in pregnancy
Antithrombin deficiency	Type 1 (quantitative)	1 in 3
	Type 2 (qualitative)	1 in 42
Factor V Leiden (FVL) homozygous		1 in 6–11
FVL heterozygous + G20210A prothrombin gene mutation heterozygous		1 in 22
Protein C deficiency		1 in 113
Protein S deficiency		1 in 113
G20210A prothrombin gene mutation heterozygous		1 in 200
FVL heterozygous		1 in 437

Deep vein thrombosis (DVT)

DVT in pregnancy: usually left-sided and proximal in the thigh or pelvis (ilio-femoral).

Clinical

- Pain and swelling of leg.
- Erythema over affected area.
- Lower abdominal pain.
- Mild pyrexia.
- Increased white cell count.

< 10% of women with clinical signs of DVT have diagnosis confirmed.

Investigations

- Imperative to confirm the diagnosis of DVT with objective testing.
- Start treatment with low molecular weight heparin (LMWH) straight away – do not wait for results of investigations.
- Can stop LMWH if diagnosis excluded.

Compression or Duplex USS leg (Doppler USS)

- Non-invasive test, first line.
- High sensitivity for femoral thromboses, not accurate for below knee DVT (which have a low tendency to cause PE).
- If Doppler USS is negative, but clinical suspicion remains, continue treatment and repeat Doppler USS in one week, or consider alternative test, e.g. venography MRI.
- If repeat testing is negative, stop treatment.

Pelvic USS with colour Doppler

- If pelvic vessel thrombosis suspected.

Magnetic resonance venography/conventional contrast venography

- Use if repeat doppler USS is negative in the presence of a strong clinical suspicion of iliac vein thrombosis (iliac fossa or back pain, swelling of the entire limb).

D-dimers

- Not useful in pregnancy.

Treatment

- Leg elevation.
- Early mobilization with graduated elastic compression stockings.
- LMWH adjusted to booking weight (see Chapter 17).

Pulmonary embolus (PE)

Symptoms
- Sudden onset pleuritic chest pain.
- Shortness of breath.
- Haemoptysis.
- Collapse or faintness.

Signs
- Tachypnoea, tachycardia.
- Raised JVP.
- Chest may sound clear.
- Symptoms and signs associated with DVT.

Differential diagnosis
- Aortic dissection.
- Chest infection.
- Intra-abdominal bleed with diaphragmatic irritation causing shoulder tip pain (abdominal signs and low JVP compared to raised JVP).

Non-diagnostic investigations

Oxygen saturation
- At rest and post-exercise: resting hypoxia, +/− fall in O_2 saturation.

CXR
- Never withold because of pregnancy: negligible radiation dose to fetus see Table 3.10.
- Mainly to exclude other pathology (e.g. pneumonia, pneumothorax, lobar collapse).
- Often initially normal or non specific.
- Subsequent abnormalities include atelectasis, consolidation, collapse, pleural effusion, elevated diaphragm, pleural basal opacities, and pulmonary oedema.

ABG
Low pO_2, low pCO_2, respiratory alkalosis.

ECG
- Mainly to exclude myocardial infarction
- Features include:
  - sinus tachycardia (usually)
  - right axis deviation
  - RBBB
  - peaked p waves in Lead II
  - S wave lead I, inverted T wave lead III, Q wave in lead I, (SI QIII TIII): rare (see Figure 16.1).

D-dimers
Do not do: unhelpful in pregnancy.

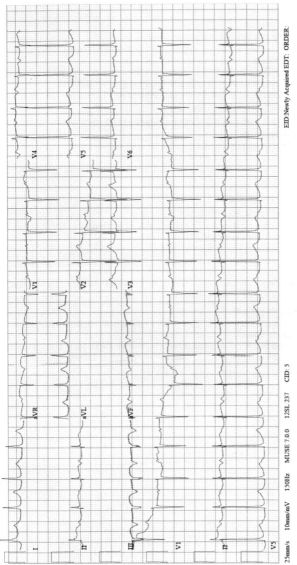

25mm/s   10mm/mV   150Hz   MUSE 7.0.0   12SL 237   CID: 5   EID:Newly Acquired EDT: ORDER:

Fig. 16.1 ECG of pregnant women with PE showing QIII, TIII, the classic full complement of SI, QIII, TIII is rarely seen.

Diagnostic investigations

Stable patient

Compression or Duplex USS legs (Doppler USS)
- If shows venous clot in legs, no further testing necessary: start treatment.
- If the Doppler negative, perform ventilation-perfusion (V/Q) lung scan or computed tomography pulmonary angiogram (CTPA).
- If tests negative, but the clinical suspicion of PE remains high, perform alternative or repeat testing.

Ventilation perfusion scan (V/Q scan) see page 52
If CXR normal:
- radiation exposure trivial: perfusion scan first:
  - if normal do not do ventilation scan
  - if abnormal do ventilation scan → treat if medium to high probability of PE.

No breast feeding for 48 hours following V/Q.

CTPA see page 50
If CXR abnormal or if V/Q not available or if the differential of aortic dissection needs exclusion:
- only detects thrombosis to level of segmental vessels
- may not detect PE in the periphery of the lungs
- less radiation to the fetus than V/Q
- significant radiation dose (2 rad) to mother (1 rad increases life time breast cancer risk by 14%).

Unstable patient
- Massive life threatening pulmonary embolus with haemodynamic compromise.
- Immediately call medical team on-call, anaesthetic team and consultant obstetrician.

See Chapter 18, p.236.

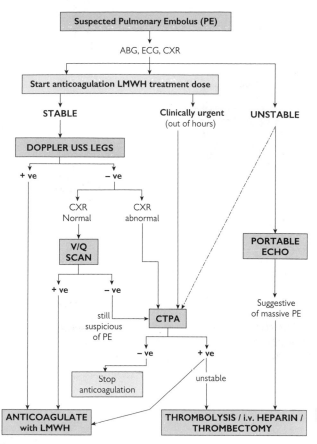

Fig. 16.2 Management of suspected pulmonary embolus in pregnancy.

Treatment

Unstable patient

E.g. collapsed/hypotensive systolic BP <90 mmHg/PaO$_2$<7 kPa. See Chapter 18, p.236.

Stable patient

- Only 5% of women with clinical signs of pulmonary embolism will have PE confirmed.
- Imperative to confirm the diagnosis of PE with objective testing.
- Before starting treatment:
  - FBC
  - coagulation screen
  - renal and liver function (heparin metabolism) may be affected if abnormal
  - thrombophilia screen: the results of this should be interpreted by clinicians (usually haematologists) with a specific expertise in this area. A limited screen for antithrombin deficiency and antiphospholipid antibodies is appropriate in pregnancy as no other thrombophilia detected will alter management
- Anticoagulate with LMWH until diagnosis excluded (see Chapter 17).

REM

Dose of LMWH in pregnancy for VTE is the same as the ACS dose, e.g. Clexane® 1 mg/kg bd NOT 1.5 mg/kg od which is the non-pregnant dose.

IVC filters

- Not recommended in pregnancy unless recurrent PE and proven DVT despite adequate anticoagulation.
- Most recurrent PE occur because of inadequate anticoagulation.

Metal valve thrombus

See Chapter 7 p.106.

Thromboprophylaxis

See Figures 16.3 and 16.4.

Assess all pregnant women for risk factors for VTE (see Table 16.1a and b):
- Before pregnancy or in early pregnancy.
- Each hospital admission.
- If have intercurrent illness.
- Immediately following delivery.

Table 16.3 Prophylactic and treatment doses of LMWH

Indication for LMWH		Enoxaparin	Dalteparin	Tinzaparin
Prophylactic dose (weight dependent)	<50 kg	20 mg od	2500 units od	3500 units od
	50–90 kg	40 mg od	5000 units od	4500 units od
	>91–130 kg	60 mg od*	7500 units od*	7000 units od*
	131–170 kg	80 mg od*	10000 units od*	9000 units od*
	> 170 kg	0.6 mg/kg/day*	75 units/kg/day*	75 u/kg/day*
Higher prophylactic (intermediate) dose (weight 50–90 kg)		40 mg bd	5000 units bd	4500 units bd
Treatment dose		1 mg/kg bd antenatal 1.5 mg/kg od postnatal	100 units/kg bd or 200 units/kg od postnatal	175 u/kg od (antenatal and postnatal)

* can split into 2 doses

Low dose aspirin

- Aspirin inhibits platelet function.
- Platelets play a small role in venous thrombosis.
- Less effective than heparin.
- Consider if patient declines heparin, or where the benefit of heparin use antenatally is unclear, e.g. to prevent paradoxical embolus with atrial septal defect.

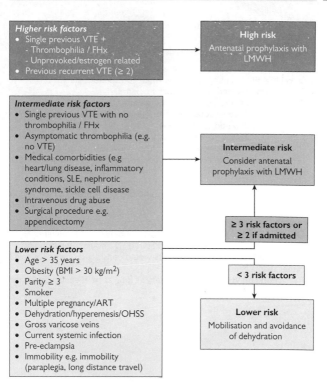

Higher risk factors
- Single previous VTE +
  - Thrombophilia / FHx
  - Unprovoked/estrogen related
- Previous recurrent VTE (≥ 2)

High risk
Antenatal prophylaxis with LMWH

Intermediate risk factors
- Single previous VTE with no thrombophilia / FHx
- Asymptomatic thrombophilia (e.g. no VTE)
- Medical comorbidities (e.g heart/lung disease, inflammatory conditions, SLE, nephrotic syndrome, sickle cell disease
- Intravenous drug abuse
- Surgical procedure e.g. appendicectomy

Intermediate risk
Consider antenatal prophylaxis with LMWH

≥ 3 risk factors or ≥ 2 if admitted

Lower risk factors
- Age > 35 years
- Obesity (BMI > 30 kg/m²)
- Parity ≥ 3
- Smoker
- Multiple pregnancy/ART
- Dehydration/hyperemesis/OHSS
- Gross varicose veins
- Current systemic infection
- Pre-eclampsia
- Immobility e.g. immobility (paraplegia, long distance travel)

< 3 risk factors

Lower risk
Mobilisation and avoidance of dehydration

Fig. 16.3 Antenatal obstetric thromboprophylaxis assessment and management.

Management of thromboprophylaxis at delivery

Induction of labour (IOL)

- Stop LMWH thromboprophylaxis 12 hours before planned IOL.

Labour

- Stop LMWH thromboprophylaxis when contractions start.
- Remain hydrated and wear support stockings.
- Regional analgesia can be used 12 hours after last dose LMWH (see Table 17.3 and see Chapter 26). If analgesia/anaesthesia required before 12 hour window:
  - in labour use alternative analgesia, e.g. opiates, fentanyl patient controlled analgesia (senior anaesthetic involvement)
  - for emergency caesarean section perform under general anaesthetic
  - Consider regional block if benefit perceived as greater than the small theoretical risk of epidural bleeding.
- Restart LMWH postnatally as long as no bleeding concerns (see Figure 16.4).

Caesarean section

- Last dose LMWH thromboprophylaxis 12 hours before delivery
- If emergency caesarean section is required <12 hours after stopping LMWH, some obstetric anaesthetists would consider a single shot spinal rather than a general anaesthetic
- Restart on LMWH evening of delivery as long as no bleeding concerns.

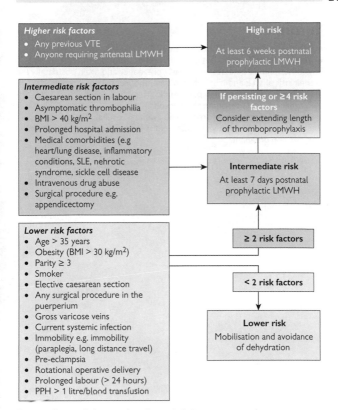

Fig. 16.4 Postnatal obstetric thromboprophylaxis assessment and management.

Summary

- Pregnancy is a prothrombotic state.
- Venous thromboembolism is a common cause of death.
- Women should be assessed in early pregnancy and again postnatally for their risk of VTE and treated with thromboprophylaxis if required.
- D-dimers are not useful in pregnancy.
- Pregnancy affects thrombophilia results.
- If VTE suspected, always treat while awaiting results of investigations.
- The dose of LMWH in VTE treatment is the ACS dose, i.e. higher than in the non pregnant.

Chapter 17

Anti-coagulation in pregnancy

Anti-coagulation in pregnancy

Indications for anticoagulation in pregnancy include:
- artificial metal heart valves
- pulmonary hypertension
- atrial fibrillation
- veno-thromboembolism (VTE) in pregnancy
- multiple previous VTE with highly thrombogenic thrombophilia.

Methods of anticoagulation:
- warfarin
- low molecular weight heparin (LMWH)
- unfractionated heparin (UH) infusion.

Table 17.1 Effects of different anticoagulants

	Warfarin	Unfractionated Heparin (UH)	Low Molecular weight Heparin (LMWH)#
Thrombosis prevention	Excellent	25% metal valve thrombosis	1% metal valve thrombosis
Crosses placenta	✓	✗	✗
Harmful effects	Embryopathy* (dose dependent)	Osteoporosis 2%	Osteoporosis 0.04%
	Fetal loss (miscarriage, IUD)	Thrombocytopenia	Injection site irritation
		Errors in administration	Allergic skin reaction 2%
	Fetal bleeding (esp. intracranial)		
Use in pregnancy	Occasional	Rare	Common
	Highly thrombogenic valve in mitral position with previous embolic event/arrythmia	If quick reversal of anticoagulation required	VTE in pregnancy
			Most metal valves
			Arrythmias
			Pulmonary hypertension
			Previous thrombosis & highly thrombogenic thrombophilia

with strict anti-Xa monitoring, dose adjustment and concomitant low dose aspirin

IUD = intrauterine death

* with use between 6–12 weeks' gestation

Warfarin

- Highly effective at preventing metal valve thrombosis and maternal death.
- Fetal embryopathy (*chondrodysplasia punctata*) in 5–6% of fetuses if used between 6–12 weeks' gestation.
- Fetal loss in one third (miscarriage, intrauterine death).
- Embryopathy and fetal loss risks are dose dependent: higher if > 5 mg used.
- Fetal bleeding especially intracranial haemorrhage with 2nd and 3rd trimester use.
- Neonatal bleeding if used at term.

Chondrodysplasia punctata, is a skeletel abnormality characterized by punctate calcification of the cartilage of the epiphyses, larynx and trachea. Symptoms include shortening of limbs and growth retardation, cataracts, dry and scaly skin and patches of coarse, dry hair. Patients may also become mildly retarded.

Low molecular weight heparin (LMWH)

- No fetal effects as does not cross placenta.
- Largely replaced warfarin for anticoagulation in pregnancy
- Most data available for enoxaparin Clexane®
- Check anti-Xa levels monthly and maintain peak levels (4 hours post dose) at:
  - 0.8–1.0 i.u/ml for aortic metal valves
  - 1.0–1.2 i.u./ml for mitral metal valves with enoxaparin
  - 0.6–0.9 i.u./ml for VTE (monitoring not usually required for acute VTE treatment).
- Monitor trough levels in high risk women also (0.4–0.7i.u./ml).
- Maternal side effects: osteoporosis 0.04%. Reversible on stopping
- Heparin induced thrombocytopenia (HIT) rare.

Table 17.2 Starting anticoagulation doses of LMWH

Enoxaparin*	Dalteparin	Tinzaparin
1 mg/kg bd antenatal	100 units/kg bd or	175 u/kg od (antenatal and postnatal)
1.5 mg/kg od postnatal**	200 units/kg od postnatal**	

* adjust dose according to anti-Xa level
** can be divided into bd dose if concern about administering large bolus dose

Unfractionated heparin

- No fetal effects as does not cross placenta.
- Requires hospital admission for continuous infusion, or ×3 subcutaneous doses/day.
- Difficult to maintain therapeutic APTT.
- 25% metal valve thrombosis rate and fetal loss rate.
- 2% incidence of maternal osteoporosis.
- Risk of heparin-induced thrombocytopenia.

Pre-pregnancy counselling

- Recommend anticoagulation after weighing up degree of risk of thrombosis with fetal risks.
- Discuss risks and benefits of different anticoagulants.
- If decision to use LMWH, then plan pregnancy and stop warfarin between 5–6 weeks' gestation to avoid embryopathy.
- If decision to continue warfarin, consider switching to LMWH between 6–12 weeks' gestation.

Antenatal care

- Multidisciplinary involvement of obstetrician, haematologist +/− cardiologist.
- If decision is to switch to LMWH, do this between 5–6 weeks' gestation:
    - monitor anti-Xa level monthly (for metal valves)
    - check calcium and Vitamin D status and replace if low.
- If warfarin is used consider switching to LMWH between 6–12 weeks' gestation:
    - maintain INR 3.0–3.5 for metal valves, INR 2.0–2.5 for other thromboses
    - monthly fetal scans
    - stop warfarin and replace with LMWH 10 days to 2 weeks pre-delivery to allow for clearance from the fetal circulation
    - for metal valves, if LMWH used, add low dose aspirin (75 mg/day) as adjunctive antithrombotic therapy.
- Put specific obstetric, anticoagulation and anaesthetic management plan for delivery in notes.

Delivery

- Aim for vaginal delivery unless obstetric indication for caesarean section.
- Management of anticoagulation depends on the importance of maintaining a given antithrombotic or anticoagulant effect.
- Women may be on prophylactic (e.g. 40 mg enoxaparin), high prophylactic (e.g. 40 mg 12 hourly enoxaparin) or fully anticoagulant doses of LMWH or warfarin.
- Risks in labour/delivery of the anticoagulated patient:
  - epidural haematoma (very rare) if regional analgesia/anaesthesia required for labour/delivery.
  - National consensus regarding timings of insertion and removal of epidural catheters see Table 17.3
  - maternal bleeding at delivery post partum haemorrhage
  - wound haematomas.
- Induction of labour may be considered to limit these risks.

Table 17.3 Cautionary use of regional analgesia techniques in pregnant women on LMWH

Regional analgesia in pregnant women on LMWH		Timing to avoid epidural haematoma
Regional analgesia can be given	On prophylactic LMWH	≥12 hours after last dose
	On therapeutic LMWH	≥24 hours after last dose
Epidural catheter removal	On LMWH	10–12 hours after last dose
	Next dose LMWH	≥3 hours after removal

Management of anticoagulation for delivery

For management of prophylactic doses of LMWH see Chapter 16, p.218.

Treatment dose LMWH

Induction of labour (IOL)

- Stop LMWH treatment 12–24 hours before commencement of IOL depending on parity and cervical Bishop score.

Labour

- Stop LMWH treatment when contractions start.
- Remain hydrated and wear support stockings or flowtron boots.
- Regional analgesia can be used 24 hours after last dose LMWH (see Table 17.3 and see Chapter 26). If analgesia/anaesthesia is required before 24 hour window:
  - in labour use alternative analgesia, e.g. opiates, fentanyl patient controlled analgesia (senior anaesthetic involvement)
  - for emergency caesarean section, perform under general anaesthesia
  - consider single shot spinal if risk of general anaesthetic is high.

Prolonged IOL/labour > 24 hours after last dose of therapeutic LMWH

Several options available – depends on degree of thrombotic risk:

- withhold heparin until after delivery – not suitable if metal valve, or if VTE less than 1 week before delivery
- further prophylactic dose of LMWH every 24 hours in labour (offer elective siting of an epidural 3 hours before each dose). Stop LMWH as soon as contractions start
- prophylactic subcutaneous UH (7500iu) 12 hourly (allows siting of an epidural after 2 hours)
- intravenous UH infusion (about 1000 units/hour) provides prophylactic levels of UH. Stop infusion at onset of the second stage of labour or interrupt it 1–2 hours prior to regional anaesthesia or analgesia.

Caesarean section

- Last dose LMWH in the morning before delivery.
- Restart LMWH thromboprophylaxis on the evening of delivery as long as there are no bleeding concerns.

Warfarin

- Many clinicians prefer to plan delivery in women on warfarin antenatally.
- There is a high risk of thrombosis when warfarin is stopped at 36 weeks and changed to LMWH or UH.
- IOL or elective caesarean section at 38 weeks minimizes the time spent off warfarin.

Unfractionated heparin (UH)

- Can be used:
  - when stopping warfarin at 36 weeks' gestation until delivery
  - when IOL or labour is prolonged > 24 hours after the last dose of therapeutic LMWH.
- Labour intensive, requires hospital admission and careful monitoring of APTT levels which can be difficult, often leading to under or over anticoagulation.

Fully anticoagulated woman on warfarin or heparin needing urgent delivery

- Reverse warfarin with fresh frozen plasma (FFP). Vitamin K (1 mg i.v.) can be used, but it usually avoided as post-partum anticoagulation with warfarin can be very difficult.
- Reverse UH with protamine sulphate. UH has a short half life and reversal is not usually required (especially not with doses of UH of 1000 U/h).
- LMWH is partially reversed with protamine sulphate.
- There is a 2% chance of wound haematoma with both LMWH and UH
- If a fully anticoagulated patient requires a caesarean section, this should be performed under general anaesthesia with insertion of wound drains and use of staples or interrupted skin sutures. This allows for early detection of bleeding.

Postnatally

- Restart LMWH thromboprophylaxis postnatally if no bleeding concerns.
- Restart LMWH treatment (anticoagulant) dose on the following day if there are no bleeding concerns (see Table 17.2)
- If there is concern about post partum haemorrhage (PPH), keep LMWH dose at high prophylactic levels until this concern passes. PPH and blood transfusion are independent risk factors for VTE
- If on long-term anticoagulation, start warfarin 5–7 days following delivery (to minimize the risk of secondary PPH).
- Continue LMWH until INR is ≥ 2 for VTE or ≥ 2.5 with mechanical valves.
- Both warfarin and LMWH are safe to use in breast feeding.

Cardiac emergencies in pregnancy

Cardiac arrest

- Occurrence: 1:30000 deliveries.
- Follow established guidelines on resuscitation from the resuscitation council (see Figure 18.1).

Differences in pregnant woman

- Resuscitate in left lateral position to prevent aortocaval compression by the pregnancy, i.e. place a wedge under the right side of the woman or tilt her pelvis to the left while keeping her torso flat to allow cardiac compressions.
- Chest compressions are more difficult due to enlarged breasts and splinting of the diaphragm.
- After 20–22 weeks' gestation, deliver the baby by caesarean section within 5 minutes of an arrest (regardless of whether the baby is still alive or not) to assist the resuscitation, i.e. delivery is to save the mother not the fetus.
- Amniotic fluid embolism and peripartum cardiomyopathy may be pregnancy related causes of cardiac arrest.

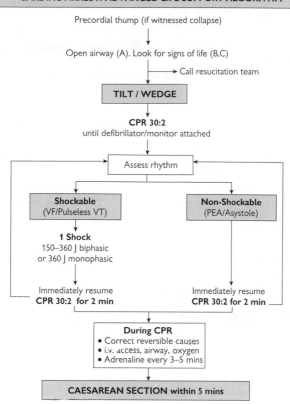

Fig. 18.1 Cardiac arrest advanced life support alogarithm in pregnancy.

Massive pulmonary embolus

See Chapter 16.

> *Unstable patient: Massive life threatening pulmonary embolus with haemodynamic compromise*
>
> e.g. collapsed/hypotensive SBP <90 mmHg / PaO_2 < 7 kPa

Differential diagnosis
- Aortic dissection.
- Myocardial infarction.
- Large intra-abdominal bleed.

Immediately call medical team on-call, anaesthetic team, consultant obstetrician and on-call cardiologist.

Investigation
See Figure 16.1:
- ABG
- ECG
- Portable CXR
- Portable echocardiogram:
  - with a large PE: evidence of right atrial or ventricular dilatation or strain
  - thrombus seen if it is very proximal in the pulmonary artery
  - helpful in the differential diagnosis of aortic dissection (aortic regurgitation).
- CTPA if patient is stable and can be moved to CT-suite.

Treatment of haemodynamically compromised PE

Depends on facilities available and severity of the cardiovascular compromise:

1. Thrombolysis: streptokinase or recombinant tissue plasminogen activator (rtPA)

- Clot dissolving treatment, (neither agent crosses placenta).
- More effective than i.v. heparin.
- rtPA dose can be repeated.
- Maternal bleeding occurs in 1–6% mainly around vascular catheter and puncture sites and the placenta.

2. Intravenous unfractionated heparin

- Regular check of APTT : keep 1.5–2 × normal.
- Less effective at reducing clot burden and improving haemodynamics rapidly compared to thrombolysis.

3. Surgery

- Pulmonary embolectomy under cardiopulmonary bypass: if the patient survives to theatre, results are excellent.
- Catheterisation of pulmonary artery with view to fragmentation of clot and improve blood flow.
- Catheter directed thrombolysis allows lower doses of thrombolytics to be used compared to systemic use (limited data).

Acute ST elevation myocardial infarction (STEMI)

(See Chapter 4, p. 69)

Cause of 26% of the cardiac deaths in pregnancy in the UK (2003–5). Increasing with rise in maternal age and obesity.

Symptoms

- Sudden onset central chest pain radiating to neck and left arm.
- Shortness of breath.
- Collapse.

In pregnancy the symptoms may be atypical such as epigastric pain, nausea, vomiting, dizziness.

Signs

- Tachycardia.
- Tachypnoea.
- Hypotension.
- Sweating.
- New onset murmur.
- Pulmonary oedema.

Differential diagnosis

- Aortic dissection.
- Pulmonary embolism.
- Perforated peptic ulcer.
- HELLP syndrome.

Diagnostic investigations

- Dynamic ECG changes on serial ECGs, e.g. ST elevation or new LBBB (see Figures 18.2 and 18.3).
- Cardiac enzymes not elevated (Troponin T or I) immediately therefore do not rely on for diagnosis. **Troponin should be checked at 12 hours post event.**

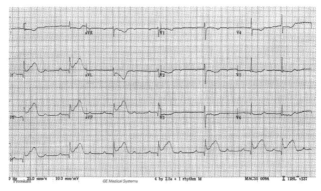

Fig. 18.2 Inferior ST elevation.

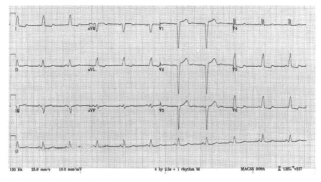

Fig. 18.3 Left Bundle Branch Block (LBBB).

Management
- Maintain oxygen saturation above 95% with Oxygen if required.
- Diamorphine 2.5–5mg IV and anti-emetic (Cyclizine, metoclopramide or prochlorperazine can be safely used).
- Coronary angiography.
- Percutaneous coronary intervention (PCI) preferable: angioplasty and or insertion of a stent (aetiology in pregnancy may be coronary artery dissection) See Chapter 4 IHD page 59.
- Thrombolysis if PCI not available.
- Care for on coronary care unit by cardiologists.

Prognosis
- Immediate maternal mortality rate between 5 and 10% and decreasing.

Aortic dissection

Cause of 19% of the cardiac deaths in pregnancy in the UK (2003–5).

Risk factors
- Marfan syndrome.
- Ehlers Danlos syndrome.
- Known aortic root dilatation.
- Hypertension.
- Bicuspid aortic valves.
- Coarctation of the aorta or surgically corrected coarctation.

Symptoms
- Sudden onset tearing chest pain radiating to back (typically interscapular).
- Shortness of breath.
- Haemoptysis.
- Collapse or faintness.

Signs
- Tachycardia.
- Tachypnoea.
- New onset aortic regurgitation murmur (diastolic at left sternal edge).
- Signs of acute MI, CVA.
- Hypotension.
- Differential BP between arms.

Differential diagnosis
- Pulmonary embolism.
- Myocardial infarction.
- Perforated peptic ulcer.

Non-diagnostic investigations
- CXR – widened mediastinum (see Figure 18.4).

Diagnostic investigations
- Echocardiogram- transoesophageal more sensitive than transthoracic.
- CT scan chest.

Management
- Ensure adequate venous access.
- Aggressive BP management, e.g. IV labetalol 40 mg bolus followed at 10 minute intervals with 40, 60, 80 mg boluses up to a maximum of 200 mg; and hydralazine 5 mg bolus repeated at 20 minute intervals up to a maximum of 20 mg. Both labetalol and hydrallazine can be given as infusions for continued control of hypertension.
- Aggressive pain relief to help reduce blood pressure, e.g. diamorphine 2.5–5mg IV plus anti-emetic.
- Further management (see Fig. 18.5).
- Fetal delivery in an emergency at < 26 weeks' gestation without having administered steroids for fetal lung maturity carries an extremely poor prognosis for the neonate.

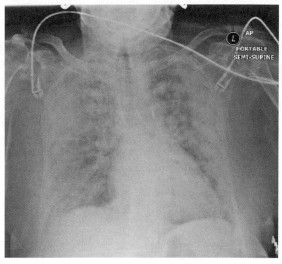

Fig. 18.4 CXR demonstrating a widened mediastinum secondary to aortic dissection.

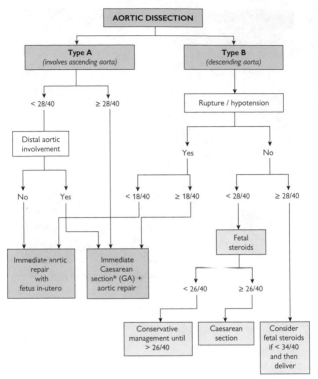

* if 18–25/40 delivery by hysterotomy or caesarean section as enlarged uterus may obstruct aortic surgery

Fig. 18.5 Management of aortic dissection in pregnancy.

Pulmonary oedema

Symptoms
- Shortness of breath, orthopnoea, paroxysmal nocturnal dyspnoea.
- Cough.
- Wheeze.
- Haemoptysis.

Signs
- Tachycardia, tachypnoea.
- Raised JVP.
- Chest auscultation: diffuse crackles, wheeze.
- Pleural effusions.

Risk factors increasing the risk
- Anaemia.
- Multiple pregnancy.

Causes
- Pre-eclampsia.
- Valvular heart disease especially mitral stenosis.
- Peripartum cardiomyopathy.
- Iatrogenic due to:
  - excess intravenous fluid administration particularly in the context of prolonged induction or augmentation of labour with syntocinon
  - tocolysis with β-agonists (e.g. ritodrine or terbutaline).
- Sepsis.
- Myocardial infarction.
- Amniotic fluid embolism.

Investigations
- ABG: reduced PaO_2 and reduced $PaCO_2$ initially
- CXR: initially normal, subsequent perihilar pulmonary infiltrates +/– pleural effusions (see Figure 18.6).

Management
- Facial O_2, +/– CPAP: aim for O_2 saturation > 95%.
- Diamorphine 2.5 mg i.v. and anti-emetic.
- Frusemide 10–40 mg i.v. initially.
- Fluid restrict.
- Identify and treat the cause.
- Intubation and ventilation if unresponsive to treatment and PaO_2 < 7 kPa or $PaCO_2$ > 6 kPa on 100% O_2.

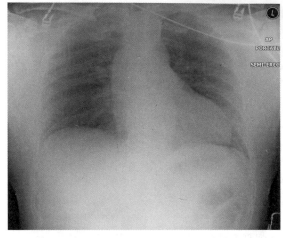

Fig. 18.6 CXR of pulmonary oedema.

Acute arrhythmias (see Chapter 9)

- Treatment as for non-pregnant with cardiac monitoring.
- Treatment usually given on CCU or ITU, but can be given on labour ward, e.g. for SVT.
- For all drug treatment have anaesthetist present and continuous fetal monitoring.
- If haemodynamic compromise use DC cardioversion.

DC cardioversion

- Any arrhythmia causing haemodynamic compromise.
- Safe at any stage in pregnancy.
- Fetus protected by amniotic fluid buffer.
- Anaesthetist may prefer intubation and ventilation.
- Keep patient on a left lateral tilt to prevent aortocaval compression
- Continuous fetal monitoring.
- Obstetrician, anaesthetist and cardiologist present.
- Proceed as in non- pregnant state.

Sustained ventricular tachycardia

- If haemodynamic compromise DC cardioversion.
- Lignocaine – drug of choice.
- β-blockers, mexiletine and procainamide can be used.
- In emergency, amiodarone can be used.

Re-entrant supraventricular tachycardia

- Vagal manoeuvres, e.g. carotid sinus massage, Valsalva manoeuvre
- Adenosine:
  - 6 mg i.v. over 2 seconds
  - if still SVT 12 mg i.v. after 1–2 mins
  - if still SVT 12 mg i.v. after 1–2 mins
  - beware of developing AV-block
- Verapamil:
  - 5 mg i.v.
  - Repeat after 5 mins if no response
- Wolff-Parkinson-White syndrome use β-blockers.

Pharmacology in pregnancy

General principles

- The physiological changes of pregnancy affect drug:
  - absorption
  - action
  - metabolism
- Greatest risk of drug-induced congenital malformations occurs during weeks 3–11 when fetal organogenesis occurs. This is complete by the end of the first trimester
- In the second and third trimester, drugs mainly affect either:
  - fetal growth
  - functional development
  - direct toxicity to the tissues
- Fetal affects are dependent upon whether the drug crosses the placenta which in turn is related to molecular size.
- On average, the fetus is exposed to no more than 10% of maternal levels.
- If drug therapy can be avoided then this should be done however, maternal risk should not be increased by withholding drugs from the mother for fear of affecting the fetus.
- A low dose should be started and then drugs uptitrated for effect.
- Mother and fetus should be monitored for drug efficacy and side effects.
- Drugs with the known proven safety profiles should be used in preference to newer drugs, i.e. the higher the FDA category (see Table 19.1) the better.

Table 19.1 FDA category

Category	Effect in pregnancy
A	Controlled studies in women fail to demonstrate a risk to the fetus in the first trimester (and there is no evidence of a risk in later trimesters), and the possibility of fetal harm appears remote.
B	Either animal-reproduction studies have not demonstrate a fetal risk but there are no controlled studies in pregnant women, or animal-reproduction studies have shown an adverse effect (other than a decrease in fertility) that was not confirmed in controlled studies in women in the first trimester (and there is no evidence of a risk in later trimesters)
C	Either studies in animals have revealed adverse effects on the fetus (teratogenic and embryocidal or other) and there are no controlled studies in women, or studies in women and animals are not available. Drugs should be given only if the potential benefit justifies the potential risk to the fetus.
D	There is positive evidence of human fetal risk, but the benefits from use in pregnant women may be acceptable despite the risk (e.g. if the drug is needed in a life-threatening situation or for a serious disease for which safer drugs cannot be used or are ineffective).
X	Studies in animals or human beings have demonstrated fetal abnormalities, or there is evidence of fetal risk based upon human experience or both, and the risk of the use of the drug in pregnant women clearly outweighs any possible benefit. The drug is contraindicated in women who are or may become pregnant.

For the management of a specific condition, please consult the relevant chapter. Table 19.2 is a quick reference guide for the common drugs used in obstetric cardiology.

Table 19.2 A quick reference guide for the common drugs used in obstetric cardiology

DRUG	USE	Can be used in pregnancy?	Major fetal & maternal side effects	Breast feeding	FDA
ACE inhibitors/ ARBs	Should only be used post-partum unless for exceptional circumstances	No	Fetal hypoperfusion, renal failure and dysgenesis Higher risk of cardiovascular and neurological congenital malformations	Yes (enalapril and captopril) ARBs – no data available	D
Adenosine	Antiarrhythmic	Yes		Yes	C
Amidoarone	Antiarrhythmic	No (unless emergency)	Congenital goitre and fetal hypo or hyperthyroidism	No	D
Amlodipine	Antihypertensive	Yes		No data available	C
Aspirin	Antiplatelet	Yes	Bleeding		C ≤ 150mg, D > 150mg
Atenolol	Hypertension, IHD, Aortic pathology, MS	Yes	Increased risk of FGR ONLY if used in first trimester. *	Yes	D
Bisoprolol	Cardioselective Beta-blocker	Yes		No data available	C

* Increased risk of IUGR ONLY if used in the first trimester.

Table 19.2 (*Contd.*) A quick reference guide for the common drugs used in obstetric cardiology

DRUG	USE	Y/N in pregnancy	Major fetal & maternal side effects	Breast feeding	FDA
Cholestyramine	Lipid lowering	Yes	Binds fat soluble vitamins therefore may result in haemorrhagic complications in utero	No data available	B
Clonidine	Anti-hypertensive occasionally used 3rd trimester for refractory HT	Yes	Hypertensive crisis if withdrawn suddenly	No data available but excreted in breast milk	C
Clopidogrel	Antiplatelet	Yes but stop before delivery	Little data	No data available	B
Digoxin	Antiarrhythmic	Yes	May need increased doses in pregnancy	Yes	C
Diltiazem	AntiHT, anti-anginal	Yes	Inadequate data Associated with increased cardiovascular defects in fetus	Yes but excreted in milk	C
Doxazosin	Third line antihypertensive	Yes		No	B

Table 19.2 (*Contd.*) A quick reference guide for the common drugs used in obstetric cardiology

DRUG	USE	Y/N in pregnancy	Major fetal & maternal side effects	Breast feeding	FDA
Fibrates	Lipid lowering	Yes	No human data or teratogenic	No	C
Flecainide	Antiarrhythmic	Yes	Proarrhythmic in mother with structural heart disease therefore avoid	Yes	C
GTN	Anti-anginal, vasodilator	Yes	Safe provided not used in very high doses	Yes	C
GIIbIIIa inhibitors	Antiplatelet	With caution	Fetal intracranial haemorrhage if given inter-partum	No data available	Tirofiban and Eptifibatide (B) Abciximab (C)
Heparin (LMWH)	Anticoagulant	Yes	Does not cross the placenta	Yes	B
Heparin (Unfractionated)	Anticoagulant	Yes	Does not cross the placenta	Yes	B
Hydralazine	2nd line antihypertensive. May be used in IV form for severe HT	Yes	S/E headache, nausea, palpitations and flushing	Yes	C
Isosorbide Mononitrate	Antianginal	Yes	Safe provided not used in very high doses	Unknown	C

Table 19.2 (*Contd.*) A quick reference guide for the common drugs used in obstetric cardiology

DRUG	USE	Y/N in pregnancy	Major fetal & maternal side effects	Breast feeding	FDA
Labetalol	Beta-blocker antihypertensive,	Yes	May provoke asthma	Yes	C
Lidocaine	Antiarrhythmic/ local anaesthetic	Yes		Yes	B
Loop Diuretics	Pulmonary congestion/ oedema	Yes		Yes but excreted in breast milk	C
Methyldopa	Beta-blocker 1st line antihypertensive	Yes	Maternal depression	Yes	B
Metoprolol	Beta-blocker IHD	Yes		Yes	C
Niacin	Lipid lowering	Yes		Excreted in breast milk therefore use doses 8-20mg only	A (C if doses above RDA used)
Nifedipine	2nd line antihypertensive	Yes	Reflex tachycardia may occur	Yes	C
Procainamide	Antiarrhythmic	Yes	May cause miscarriage if used in high doses	Yes	C
Propafenone	Antiarrhythmic		Very little data available in pregnancy	No	C

Table 19.2 (*Contd.*) A quick reference guide for the common drugs used in obstetric cardiology

DRUG	USE	Y/N in pregnancy	Major fetal & maternal side effects	Breast feeding	FDA
Propranolol	Beta-blocker Anti-arrhythmic	Yes		Yes	C
Quinidine	Antiarrhythmic	Yes		Yes	C
Sotalol	Antiarrhythmic	Yes	Risk of torsade in mother	Yes	B
Spironolactone	AntiHT, post MI with LVSD heart failure	Yes	Antiandrogenic effects in fetus and FGR	No	D
Statins	Lipid lowering	No	Teratogenic	No	X
Thiazide diuretics	HT	Yes			D
Thrombolytics	Alteplase	Yes	Placental bleeding	Unknown	C
Verapamil	Antiarrhythmic	Yes	Rapid IV may precipitate maternal hypotension	Yes but excreted in milk	C
Warfarin	Anticoagulant	No in first trimester* and at time of delivery/ caution in rest of pregnancy	Warfarin embryopathy, fetal intracranial haemorrhage intra uterine death	Yes	X

* between 6 to 12 weeks gestation

Beta-blockers in pregnancy

- Concern about FGR in pregnancy evolved from their use as antihypertensives for hypertensive disorders in pregnancy, i.e. pre-eclampsia (PET).
- PET is associated with FGR due to abnormal placentation even when atenolol is not used.
- Cochrane review suggests concern over beta-blockers remains with atenolol but only when given in the first trimester.
- **Atenolol when commenced in the 2nd or 3rd trimesters does not appear to be associated with FGR.**
- **Women needing atenolol in pregnancy, i.e. Marfan patient, should be given it despite concerns over FGR and serial growth scans carried out on the baby.**
- Increasing experience with newer cardioselective beta-blockers metoprolol and bisoprolol has been gained and appears safe although higher doses may be required in pregnancy.

Antibiotics with adverse effects during pregnancy

- Aminoglycosides – ototoxicity and fetal deafness, though this is not a problem if drug levels are monitored.
- Chloramphenicol – Grey baby syndrome and haemolysis in women or fetus with G6PD deficiency.
- Sulphonamides – neonatal jaundice if given > 34 weeks' gestation.
- Tetracycline – Slowed bone growth and enamel hypoplasia.
- Trimethoprim – Neural tube defects if used in 1st trimester.

The multidisciplinary team management of heart disease in pregnancy

The multidisciplinary team

Cardiac disease in pregnancy is now the leading cause of maternal death in the UK.

Substandard care and poor communication between different specialities are significant contributing causes to this maternal mortality.

Multidisciplinary management with a team of doctors, midwifery and nursing staff is imperative to ensure appropriate care of the mother and her fetus in order to lead to the most favourable outcomes.

The multidisciplinary team includes:
- obstetrician, with expertise in maternal medicine
- cardiologist, with expertise in obstetric cardiology
- obstetric physician
- obstetric anaesthetist
- neonatologist
- maternal medicine midwife
- specialist cardiology nurse.

Other teams may be involved including intensivists and different cardiologists may be required depending upon the particular cardiac condition, e.g. pulmonary hypertension experts, adult congenital heart disease consultants.

There may be conflict between the best form of management to optimise outcome of the mother and that of the baby.

Maternal health takes priority over the fetus

The outcome will not always be favourable, but difficult decisions may need to be made with input of all members of the multidisciplinary team.

The obstetrician/maternal medicine specialist

A consultant obstetrician under whose care the patient usually is:
- will monitor both maternal and fetal condition during pregnancy
- will decide the best timing and mode of delivery.

The obstetric physician

A consultant physician trained in the management of all medical disorders in pregnancy.

Can coordinate discussions between all team members and advise of specific considerations with respect to management of cardiac disease in pregnancy.

The obstetric anaesthetist

A consultant anaesthetist trained in the management of analgesia and anaesthetic requirements in pregnant women:
- will assist in fluid management, maternal monitoring, and resuscitation
- will decide whether a regional anaesthetic (spinal, epidural or combined spinal epidural) is appropriate for delivery
- will decide on appropriate postnatal analgesia.

The neonatologist

A consultant neonatologist will provide care for the neonate following delivery:

- will advise the team on likely neonatal outcomes at differing gestations
- will counsel mother regarding prognosis, specifically survival and disability statistics.

The maternal medicine midwife

A midwife who is involved in providing care to women with high risk pregnancies and with medical disorders in pregnancy:

- will provide emotional support to the mother and acts as the patient's advocate.

Royal College of Obstetricians and Gynaecologists (RCOG) recommendations (summarized)

All women of reproductive age with congenital or acquired heart disease should:

1. Have access to specialised multidisciplinary pre-conception counselling where advice on safe and effective contraception is available.
2. Receive advice from the multidisciplinary team before assisted conception is undertaken.
3. Be assessed clinically as soon as possible after conceiving by the multidisciplinary team and appropriate investigations (e.g. echo, MRI) undertaken.
4. Have appropriate care arranged at a district general hospital or tertiary centre depending on the complexity of the heart disease, risk assessment and locally available facilities and expertise.
5. Undergo risk stratification by the multidisciplinary team to determine the frequency and content of antenatal care.
6. Have intrapartum care supervised by a team experienced in the care of women with heart disease.
7. Have a clear management plan for labour and the puerperium
8. Plan for a vaginal delivery unless there are obstetric or specific cardiac considerations.
9. Have high-level multidisciplinary maternal surveillance following delivery when most of the haemodynamic changes are occurring.
10. Have multidisciplinary follow-up assessment at least 6 weeks post-natally.

Epidemiology of heart disease in pregnancy

Maternal mortality

- Cardiac disease is the leading cause of maternal death in the UK.
- There were 48 deaths due to cardiac disease between 2003–2005 in the UK.
- Maternal mortality from heart disease has been rising since the 1980s.
- Maternal death from congenital heart disease is stable (fell in 2003–2005) see Figure 21.1.
- Rise of cardiac deaths is due to an increase in acquired heart disease: most deaths are in those not previously diagnosed with heart disease.
- Congenital heart disease (CHD): 85% of infants with CHD survive to adulthood.
- 50% of all aortic dissections in women < 40 years occur in pregnancy.

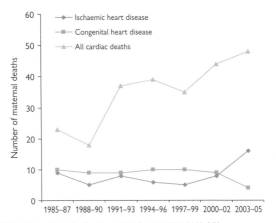

Fig. 21.1 Maternal deaths due to cardiac disease 1985–2005, UK.

- Main causes of cardiac-related maternal deaths in the UK:
  - myocardial infarction: mainly due to ischaemic heart disease (IHD)
  - aortic dissection: mainly thoracic aorta
  - cardiomyopathy: mainly peripartum (PPCM).
- Other cardiac causes of maternal death:
  - Sudden Adult Death Syndrome (SADS)
  - myocarditis/myocardial fibrosis
  - valvular heart disease
  - infectious endocarditis
  - RV/LV hypertrophy or hypertensive heart failure
  - pulmonary hypertension
  - congenital heart disease.
- Main causes of cardiac-related maternal deaths in the developing world:
  - rheumatic heart disease.

Maternal age

- Average age of childbirth is rising in the UK.
- 1985–2005: maternities in women (Figure 21.2):
  - aged > 35 years increased from 8% to 19%
  - aged 20 to 29 years fell from 64% to 44%
- Maternal death rate rises with age: 3 × higher in women > 40 years compared to women <25 years.
- Risk of hypertension 4–9 times higher age 40 compared to age 20–29 years.
- Risk of MI 4.5 higher age ≥ 40 compared to 21–25 years.

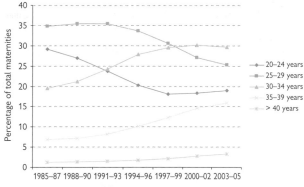

Fig. 21.2 Maternity rates 1985–2005, UK.

Ischaemic heart disease (IHD)

See Chapter 4.

- Increasing incidence of myocardial infarction in pregnant women:
  - 1991: 1.4/100000 maternities
  - 2001: 4.1/100000 maternities
  - 2002: 6.2/100000 maternities (3–4 times higher than general population).
- Due to:
  - increased detection of previously undetected small events through troponin testing
  - rising maternal age of pregnant women who have more cardiovascular risk factors, e.g. hypertension, obesity, diabetes, and pre-eclampsia
- Case fatality rates fallen from 37% in older studies to 5.1% in 2002 due to developments in diagnosis and treatment:
  - Increased cardiac catheterisation
  - Increased angioplasty instead of thrombolysis for acute MI
  - Insertion of stents.

Congenital heart disease (CHD)

- 1% of livebirths have CHD.
- Increasing survival of children born with CHD into adulthood (approximately 85%) due to improved surgical techniques and paediatric intensive care.
- Estimate of annual increase in numbers of CHD cases = 1,600.
- 800 new cases/year require specialist follow up.
- Female children with complex CHD surviving into adulthood: may wish to conceive.
- Risk of baby with CHD is increased in women with CHD to 5%.

Pre-pregnancy counselling

Pre-pregnancy counselling

Most women want to conceive and have a family. Women with heart disease are no different, but pregnancy may hold risks for the:
- Mother – disease exacerbation, cardiac decompensation, and maternal death.
- Fetus – malformations (genetic, warfarin), in-utero growth restriction, preterm delivery, stillbirth, neonatal morbidity, and mortality.

Pre-pregnancy counselling will inform women of their risks, empowering them to make an informed decision as to whether or not to proceed with pregnancy. It will allow planning or prevention of pregnancy, and access to the appropriate multidisciplinary specialized services.

Who needs it?
- Women with congenital heart disease (CHD) – 0.8% of pregnant women.
- Women with acquired heart disease – 0.1% of pregnant women.

When do they need it?
Complex congenital heart disease
- During adolescence (aged 12–15 years old) depending on degree of maturity.
- Average age of first sexual intercourse is 16 years.
- Britain has the highest rate of teenage pregnancy in Europe (6%).
- 1 in 133 girls under the age of 16 years get pregnant.

Acquired heart disease
- Following diagnosis.

Who should do it?
- Cardiologist with a special interest in pregnancy and/or
- obstetric physician.
- May also need advise from maternal medicine specialist.

What does it cover?
- Risk assessment: with full history, examination and investigations as appropriate (e.g. ECG, echocardiogram, MRI).
- Consideration of effects of the cardiac disease on pregnancy:
  - maternal risks
  - fetal risks.
- Consideration of effects of the pregnancy on the cardiac disease:
  - risk of deterioration
  - effect of treatment or intervention in pregnancy in event of deterioration
  - mortality risk.

- Discussion as to whether pregnancy should be contemplated, delayed or avoided.
- Prevention/delay of pregnancy with the most appropriate contraceptive agent.
- Preparation for pregnancy if this is considered appropriate.
- Other methods of having a family if pregnancy is not recommended:
  - surrogacy
  - adoption.
- If maternal life expectancy is limited, discussion on appropriateness of having a baby (by pregnancy, surrogacy or adoption) and issues of child-care in the event of maternal mortality or severe morbidity.
- Long-term prognosis following pregnancy: despite one successful pregnancy, some conditions have a high recurrence risk (e.g. peripartum cardiomyopathy) and others can deteriorate with age, increasing the risk to future pregnancies.
- Referral to geneticist where there is definite or suspected inherited heart disease or chromosomal abnormality.

Assessment of maternal cardiac risk

Depends on establishing:
1. maternal functional status (from history – see Table 22.1)
2. the underlying cardiac lesion see Table 22.2
3. need for further corrective/palliative surgery
4. additional associated risk factors, e.g. anticoagulation.

Table 22.1 New York Heart Association (NYHA) functional classification

NYHA Class	Description
I	No breathlessness/uncompromised
II	Breathlessness on severe exertion/slightly compromised
III	Breathlessness on mild exertion/moderately compromised
IV	Breathlessness at rest/severely compromised

Table 22.2 Underlying cardiac lesion

Class 1	No contraindications to pregnancy: no detectable increased risk	
	Uncomplicated, small or mild lesions	Mitral valve prolapse with trivial mitral regurgitation
		Patent ductus arteriosus
		Ventricular septal defect
	Successfully repaired simple lesions	Patent ductus arteriosus
		Ventricular septal defect
		Ostium secundum atrial septal defect
		Total anomalous pulmonary venous drainage
	Isolated ventricular extrasystoles and atrial ectopic beats	
Class 2	Can consider pregnancy: small increased risk (< 1% maternal death or severe disability)	
	if well and uncomplicated	Unoperated atrial septal defect
		Repaired tetralogy of Fallot
		Arrythmias

Table 22.2 (*Contd.*) Underlying cardiac lesion

Class 2–3	Depending on individual	Mild left ventricular impairment
		Hypertrophic cardiomyopathy
		Native or tissue valvular heart disease not considered class 4 congenital heart disease
		Marfan syndrome without aortic dilatation
		Heart transplantation
Class 3	**Requires expert counselling: significantly increased risk Intensive specialist cardiac and obstetric monitoring in pregnancy and post-partum**	
		Mechanical heart valve
		Systemic right ventricle
		Post Fontan operation (for tricuspid atresia)
		Cyanotic heart disease
		Other complex congenital heart disease
Class 4	**Pregnancy not advisable: high risk of serious maternal morbidity or mortality Emergency contraception /termination of pregnancy. If declined, care for as Class 3**	
	Pulmonary arterial hypertension	Any cause
	Severe systemic ventricular dysfunction with either	NYHA III-IV
		Left ventricular ejection fraction < 30%
	Previous peripartum cardiomyopathy	With any residual impairment of left ventricular function
	Severe left heart obstruction	Aortic/ mitral stenosis with valve area < 1 cm^2
	Marfan syndrome	With aortic dilatation > 4 cm
	Women with ≥ 2 of the following risk factors	Impaired left ventricular function with ejection fractions < 40%
		Left heart obstruction:
		aortic stenosis with valve area < 1.5 cm^2
		mitral stenosis with valve area < 2 cm^2
		Previous cardiovascular events, e.g. heart failure, transient ischaemic attacks or stroke
		NYHA ≥ II

One can predict the risk of a significant cardiac event in pregnancy using the *Toronto risk score*.

Toronto risk predictor score

Establish whether the following criteria are present. Each separate point is one predictor:
- Previous episode of heart failure, transient ischaemic attack, cerebrovascular accident or arrhythmia
- NYHA ≥ II or cyanosis
- Left heart obstruction:
  - mitral valve area < 2 cm^2 or
  - aortic valve area < 1.5 cm^2 or
  - peak left ventricular outflow tract obstruction > 30 mmHg on echo
- reduced left ventricular function (ejection fraction < 40%).

Toronto risk predictor score

Number of predictors	Risk of a cardiac event in pregnancy
0	5%
1	27%
≥ 2	75%

Assessment of fetal risk

- Congenital malformations due to teratogenesis:
  - 6% warfarin embryopathy when used between 6–12 weeks' gestation
  - 6% with use of angiotensin converting enzyme (ACE) inhibitors in the first trimester.
- Inherited fetal cardiac malformations (typically 3%, but varies according to which the parent affected, the specific lesion (higher with left sided lesions), and the number of offspring previously affected see Tables 22.3 and 22.4). Fetal echocardiography would be performed in the second trimester.
- Inherited syndromes such as Marfan syndrome (autosomal dominant): discuss recurrence risk (50%), postnatal follow-up of baby and long-term surveillance.
- Fetal growth restriction: with cyanotic heart disease, use of beta-blockers.
- Prematurity (iatrogenic due to preterm delivery) with associated neonatal morbidity and mortality. The risk is related to the gestation at delivery (see Table 22.5).
- Stillbirth secondary to maternal cyanosis (see Table 22.6) or warfarin use.

Table 22.3 Risk of congenital heart disease (CHD)

Risk factor	Risk CHD in future pregnancy (%)
Father with CHD	2
Mother with CHD	5
One previous child with CHD	2
Two previous children with CHD	10

Table 22.4 Risk of congenital heart disease (CHD) in offspring of an affected parent

Specific CHD in parent		Risk in offspring* (%)
Intracardiac shunts	Atrial septal defect	3–11
	Ventricular septal defect	4–22
	Patent ductus arteriosus	4–11
Outflow obstruction	Left-sided**	3–26
	Right-sided	3–22
	Hypertrophic cardiomyopathy	50
Complex abnormalities	Tetralogy of Fallot	4–15

*same or related lesion
**including coarctation of the aorta and congenital aortic stenosis (sub-, valvular and supravalvular)

Table 22.5 Neonatal survival at very early gestations

Gestation at delivery (completed)	Neonatal survival
23 weeks	11%
24 weeks	26%
25 weeks	44%

Of the survivors, by age 6 years, between 25–46% (depending on addition of cognitive measures to physical disability) do not function within the normal range, or have a disability which would prevent them from being independent.

Table 22.6 Livebirth rates with varying degrees of cyanosis

Maternal oxygen saturation (%)	Livebirth rate (%)
> 90	92
≥ 85–90	63
< 85	12

Preparation for pregnancy

Once risk assessment has been performed, it is ultimately the woman's decision, based on informed choice, as to whether or not to proceed with pregnancy. The clinician's duty is to ensure that she has been fully informed and counselled in order to make that decision. Even if she has a condition in class 4 of Table 22.2, i.e. a condition where pregnancy is not recommended, if she decides to proceed with pregnancy, she should be assured that the multidisciplinary team will care for her to the best of their ability and without judgement.

The key aims are to ensure that the woman is as healthy as possible to proceed with pregnancy, with the best cardiac function that can be achieved and that any medications she is taking are appropriate for pregnancy. The following should be assessed and procedures performed prior to pregnancy:

- Mitral or aortic stenosis e.g. valve area <2 cm^2 or 1.5 cm^2 respectively consider:
  - valvotomy (open or closed)
  - valve replacement if valvotomy not suitable – careful consideration as to whether a tissue or mechanical valve is used as the risks of anticoagulation in future pregnancies with mechanical valves need to be balanced against their greater durability compared to tissue valves (see Chapter 7).
- Arrythmias: define with Holter monitoring and treat medically or surgically e.g. surgical ablation or radio frequency of an accessory pathway in Wolff-Parkinson White syndrome (see Chapter 14).
- Dilated aortic root, e.g. ≥ 4 cm^2: aortic root repair.
- Previous surgical repair: assess to ensure there are no sequelae, e.g.:
  - aortic coarctation repair with Dacron graft – echocardiogram and aortic MRI to identify any re-stenosis and exclude post stenotic dilatation or aneurysm formation
  - previous valve repair/replacement and complex CHD repair echocardiogram to assess repair and ventricular function and exclude atrial or ventricular dilatation.
- Underlying medical conditions: e.g. optimise control of hypertension with non-teratogenic medication (avoid ACE inhibitors); optimize diabetic control.
- Anticoagulation: continue warfarin until 6 weeks' gestation. Discussion as to whether it is appropriate to change to low molecular weight heparin after 6 weeks to avoid warfarin embryopathy, miscarriage, fetal intracranial haemorrhage, and still birthrisks with ongoing warfarin use. This is to be balanced against risks of thrombosis (see Chapter 21).
- Avoidance of teratogenic medication, e.g. ACE inhibitors.
- Dental treatment: if complex CHD should have dental work performed pre-pregnancy in a hospital department.

- Obesity risks: aim for a normal BMI to reduce risks in pregnancy.
- General pre-pregnancy advice including cessation of smoking, take 0.4 mg of periconceptional folic acid from when starting to try for pregnancy until 12 weeks' pregnant, to reduce the risk of fetal neural tube defects.
- Contact information: to contact multidisciplinary team as soon as pregnancy is confirmed.

Maternal age at pregnancy

Increasing maternal age results in:
- reduced fertility
- increased need for assisted reproductive technologies to conceive
- increase in miscarriage rates
- increase in fetal chromosomal abnormalities
- increase in adverse pregnancy outcomes.

Reduced fertility and increase in miscarriage rates

As women get older they will find it more difficult to conceive. If they do conceive they have a higher rate of miscarriage (Figure 22.1)

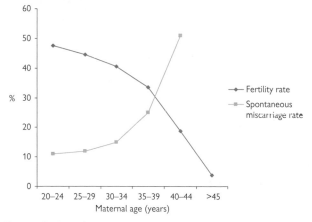

Fig. 22.1 Fertility and miscarriages rates with maternal age.

Increased need for assisted reproductive technologies to conceive

More older women will opt for assisted reproductive techniques to get pregnant as their fertility declines. This carries additional risks to the woman with heart disease that should be discussed before committing to these procedures. The risks include:

- Ovarian hyperstimulation resulting in large fluid shift into the third space, intravascular fluid depletion and thrombosis.
- Multiple pregnancies which increase the risk of diabetes and hypertensive disease in pregnancy as well as having a greater effect on cardiac function.

Increase in fetal chromosomal abnormalities

All fetal chromosomal abnormalities increase with maternal age (see Table 22.7). The commonest is Down's syndrome, Trisomy 21.

Table 22.7 Risk of Down's syndrome with maternal age

Maternal Age (years)	Risk of chromosomal abnormality	Risk of Down's syndrome
15–24	1/500	1/1500
25–29	1/385	1/1100
35	1/178	1/350
40	1/63	1/100
45	1/18	1/25

Prenatal diagnosis should be discussed, both screening and definitive tests and an explanation given of their risks and accuracy (see Chapter 5). Options for termination of pregnancy or continuation of pregnancy in the event of an affected fetus should be discussed with the parents.

Increase in adverse pregnancy outcomes

All adverse pregnancy outcomes, both maternal and fetal, increase with maternal age. Figure 22.2 shows the risk of maternal death with increasing age. It is preferable for women to conceive in their twenties and early thirties to minimize these risks. This is particularly true for women with medical diseases like heart disease, where the development of, e.g. hypertension or diabetes in pregnancy due to maternal age may have a greater impact on their cardiac status. If a woman is in a position to make a judgement as to the timing of her pregnancy, she should be encouraged not to delay it until her late thirties to forties.

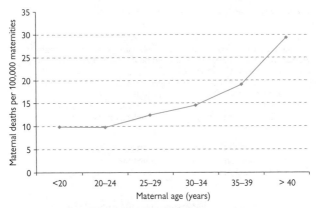

Fig. 22.2 Maternal deaths by age 2003–5, UK (data from Confidential enquiry into maternal and child deaths: CEMACH).

Diversity and beliefs

In a multicultural society there will be couples who hold a variety of opinions or beliefs which need to be respected. These will be shaped by religious, cultural, and social contexts. Counselling should encompass all the points above but the clinician should be aware of specific issues, e.g.:

- religious beliefs relating to contraception and termination of pregnancy
- importance given to the partner's and extended family's opinion in some cultures
- language barriers – where the woman may not speak or fully understand English. It is imperative to have an interpreter in these situations and not rely on the partner, family, or friend to interpret as they may have a different opinion and not pass on all the information in an unbiased manner.

Contraception

Introduction

Contraceptive agents are used to prevent pregnancy. No method is completely effective. Efficacy depends on the method used and user-compliance. The most efficacious contraceptives are long acting agents and surgical methods which do not rely on the user (Table 23.1).

Table 23.1 Failure rates of contraceptives

Contraceptive method	% of women experiencing an unintended pregnancy within first year of typical use
No method	85
Spermicides	29
Withdrawal	27
Periodic abstinence	25
Barriers (cap, sponge, diaphragm, condoms)	15–32
COC and POP	8
Combined hormonal patch (Evra®)	8
Combined hormonal (NuvaRing®)	8
DMPA (Depo-Provera®)	3
Combined injectable (Lunelle™)	3
Copper T IUD	0.8
Mirena® (LNG-IUS)	0.1
Female sterilisation	0.5
Male sterilisation	0.15
Implant (Implanon®)	0.05

COC = combined oral contraceptive pill; POP = progesterone-only pill
LNG-IUS = levonorgestrel intra-uterine system

Combined hormonal contraceptives

- Combinations of oestradiol and a progestogen which inhibit ovulation.
- The most common form of contraception used by women.
- Available as a pill (combined oral contraceptive pill: COC pill), skin patch, or vaginal ring.

Advantages

- Efficaceous.
- Menstrual cycle regularity and lighter periods.

Disadvantages

Increased risk of the following due to oestrogen:

- Arterial thrombosis—ischaemic stroke, ischaemic heart disease especially if other risk factors are present, e.g. smoking, hypertension, diabetes, obesity.
- Venous thrombosis—3rd generation COC have a higher risk than 2nd generation COC:
  - embolic stroke from deep vein thrombosis if patent foramen ovale (PFO) or right-to-left shunt
- Cardiac thrombosis despite anticoagulation if mechanical heart valves, atrial fibrillation or cardiomyopathy (dilated/peripartum).
- Interaction with warfarin—monitor INR more frequently.

See Tables 23.2 and 23.3 for relative and absolute contraindications.

Table 23.2 Absolute contraindications for using combined hormonal contraception

System	Disease
Arterial	Severe hypertension untreated: SBP ≥160 mmHg or DBP ≥95 mmHg
	Hypertension with vascular disease*
	Ischaemic heart disease
	Cerebrovascular accident
	Complicated valvular and congenital heart disease**
	Multiple risk factors for cardiovascular disease#
Venous	Thrombosis (deep vein thrombosis, pulmonary embolism or cerebral venous thrombosis)
	Major surgery with prolonged immobilization
	Known thrombophilia
Endocrine	Diabetes mellitus >20 years
	Diabetes mellitus with severe vascular disease or severe nephropathy, retinopathy or neuropathy
Breast	Breastfeeding < 6 weeks post-partum
	Current breast cancer
Metabolic	Obesity ≥ 40 kg/m² BMI
Neurological	Migraine with aura
	Migraine without aura and age ≥ 35 years *(C)*
Liver	Active viral hepatitis
	Severe (decompensated) cirrhosis
	Benign or malignant liver tumours
Connective Tissue	Systemic lupus erythematosus with anticardiolipin antibodies/lupus anticoagulant
Drugs	Smoking ≥15 cigarettes/day and age ≥ 35 years

* coronary heart disease, peripheral vascular disease, hypertensive retinopathy, transient ischaemic attacks
** e.g. with pulmonary hypertension, atrial fibrillation, history of bacterial endocarditis
#age, smoking, diabetes mellitus, hypertension, hyperlipidaemia
BMI = body mass index; *C* = continuation of contraceptive

Table 23.3 Relative contraindications for using combined hormonal contraception

System	Disease
Arterial	Adequately controlled hypertension
	Moderate hypertension untreated: SBP <160mmHg or DBP <95 mmHg
	Multiple risk factors for arterial disease
Venous	First-degree relative age < 45 years with VTE
	Immobility unrelated to surgery
Endocrine	Diabetes mellitus with mild/moderate vascular disease/nephropathy/retinopathy/neuropathy
Breast	Not breastfeeding < 3 weeks post-partum
	Fully breastfeeding ≥6 weeks to 6 months post-partum
	Breast cancer > 5 years ago without recurrence
	Carriers of known gene mutations associated with breast cancer
Metabolic	Some known hyperlipidaemias*
	Obesity 35–39 kg/m^2 BMI
Neurological	Previous migraine with aura at any age
	Migraine without aura age ≤ 35 years (C)
	Migraine without aura age ≥ 35 years (I)
Liver	Current or medically treated gallbladder disease
	Previous cholestasis due to combined oral contraceptives
	Obstetric cholestasis
	Mild cirrhosis (compensated)
Drugs	Liver enzyme inducers**
	Smoking <15 cigarettes/day and age ≥ 35 years
	Stopped smoking < 1 year ago

VTE = venothromboembolism; BMI = body mass index
C = continuation of contraceptive; I = initiation of contraceptive
*e.g. Familial hypercholesterolaemia; **reduces contraceptive effectiveness

Progestogen-only contraceptives

- Generally safer than combined hormonal contraceptives as do not contain oestrogen.
- Better choice in women with heart disease.

Available as:
- Mini-pills (progesterone-only pills (POP)):
  - standard POP—this must be taken at the same time each day
  - Cerazette®—this is anovulatory and more effective
- Injection (Depo-Provera).
- Intra-uterine device (Mirena®: levonorgestrel [LNG] IUS).
- Subcutaneous implant (Implanon®).

Advantages
- Reduced menstrual blood loss with continued use, which is particularly beneficial if:
  - on warfarin which causes menorrhagia
  - cyanotic heart diease—less anaemia (more important for those women who are not polycythaemic)
- Use in many cases where COC contraindicated.

Disadvantages
- Irregular menstrual bleeding.
- Interacts with warfarin metabolism—monitor INR more frequently.
- Reduced contraceptive efficacy of POP and Implanon® with bosentan (enzyme inducer).

Depo-provera
- Intramuscular injection lasts for 12 weeks.
- Haematoma can occur at injection site if anticoagulated.
- Hypo-oestrogenic status with long term use: may not be appropriate in women with ischaemic heart disease.

Mirena IUS
- Insertion into uterus and releases levonorgestrel directly into uterus with little systemic absorption.
- Cover insertion with antibiotics
  - empirically if not screened for sexually transmitted infections
  - if at risk of bacterial endocarditis
- Effective for 5 years.
- More effective than sterilisation.
- Insertion can cause bradycardia from vagal stimulation—avoid in women with pulmonary hypertension or Fontan circulation or fit in hospital with anaesthetist present.

Implanon

- Inserted into subdermal tissue of non-dominant arm under local anaesthetic.
- Remove and replace after 3 years.
- If used in the anticoagulated patient, apply prolonged pressure after insertion.

See Table 23.4 for relative contraindications to progesterone-only contraception.

Table 23.4 Relative contraindications for using progestogen-only methods of contraception

System	Disease
Arterial	Hypertension with vascular disease *(Injectables)*
	Multiple risk factors for cardiovascular disease* *(Injectables)*
	Ischaemic heart disease *(Injectables; POP/IMP I/C)*
	Cerebrovascular accident *(Injectables; POP/IMP I/C)*
Venous	Current thrombosis on anticoagulation (deep vein thrombosis, pulmonary embolism or cerebral venous thrombosis) *(Injectables/IMP)*
Endocrine	Diabetes mellitus >20 years *(Injectables)*
	Diabetes mellitus with vascular disease ie nephropathy, retinopathy or neuropathy *(Injectables)*
Breast	Breastfeeding < 6 weeks post-partum
	Breast cancer > 5 years ago without recurrence
Neurological	Migraine with aura *(all methods: C)*
Liver	Active viral hepatitis
	Severe (decompensated) liver cirrhosis
	Tumours: benign/malignant liver tumours
Drugs	Liver enzyme inducers *(POP/IMP)*

* age, smoking, diabetes mellitus, hypertension, hyperlipidaemia
I = initiation of contraceptive
C = continuation of contraceptive
POP = progesterone-only pill
IMP = implant

Copper intrauterine contraceptive device (Copper IUD)

- Inserted into the uterus after cervical dilatation, usually as an outpatient
- Cover insertion with antibiotics:
  - empirically if not screened for sexually transmitted infections
  - if at risk of bacterial endocarditis
- Replace after 5–10 years.

Advantages

- Non-hormonal
- Effective.

Disadvantages

- Infection during insertion and with long-term use:
  - avoid in women with previous bacterial endocarditis
  - caution if complicated valvular disease
- Bradycardia with insertion due to cervical dilatation (less common than with Mirena®).
- Menorrhagia—caution if anticoagulated.

Sterilisation

- Considered irreversible.
- Failure rate—not the most efficaceous contraceptive.
- Regret.
- Only to be considered if family is complete, or if patient advised against pregnancy.

Female sterilisation

Surgical occlusion of both fallopian tubes at:

- Laparoscopy—commonest method, under general anaesthetic, Filshie clips applied to each fallopian tube; failure rate 1:200.
- Mini-laparotomy.
- Caesarean section (CS)—removal of part of both fallopian tubes; failure rate 1:100. Removal of both fallopian tubes (salpingectomies) can be considered at time of CS in cases where further pregnancy is not recommended, e.g. pulmonary hypertension.
- Hysteroscopy with ESSURE—intratubal insertion of stents into the proximal part of fallopian tubes, under local or general anaesthetic.

Advantages

- Efficaceous.

Disadvantages

- Usually requires a general anaesthetic.
- Failure rate 1:100–1:200 depending on method used
- Relative increase in ectopic pregnancies in failures.
- Regret.
- Laparoscopy involves insufflation of peritoneum with CO_2:
  - reduces venous return → contraindicated in pulmonary hypertensives and those with Fontan circulation
  - systemic absorption CO_2 → paradoxical emboli if right-to-left shunt
- ESSURE®
  - Bradycardia from vagal stimulation during insertion of hysteroscope in 1.85%
  - Tubal occlusion takes 3 months.

Male sterilisation

- Surgical occlusion of vas deferens under local anaesthetic.
- Sterility confirmed with two sperm-free specimens at 3–4 months post-operatively.
- Failure rate 1.5/1000.
- Safest form of contraception for women.
- Avoid in partners of women with severe heart disease who have a reduced life span.

Emergency contraception

For women who failed to take appropriate precautions against pregnancy, i.e. unprotected sexual intercourse (UPSI).

Methods

Within 72 hours of UPSI

- Levonorgestrel (1.5 mg Levonelle One Step®; 0.75 mg 2 tablets Levonelle-2):
  - well tolerated in all women with heart disease
  - no medical contraindications to use
  - 1% failure rate if used within 72 hours UPSI
  - common side effects are nausea and vomiting
  - caution if on warfarin (can cause INR to increase up to 4-fold)
  - increase dose if on liver enzyme inducing drugs
- Combined oestrogen-progestogen (Yuzpe) regimen (available in some countries) within 72 hours of UPSI
  - May be more appropriate in patients anticoagulated with warfarin.
- Neither intended to be used as a regular form of contraception due to high annual failure rate.

Within 5 days of UPSI

- Copper IUD (see p.300):
  - Preferred option for women using liver enzyme inducers.

Barrier methods

Male and female condoms, caps, and diaphragms are not very effective methods for prevention of pregnancy, but should be used to prevent sexually transmitted infections in combination with a more secure contraceptive method.

Termination of pregnancy

Urgent termination of pregnancy facilities should be readily available and accessible for women with medical conditions where pregnancy places their lives at risk.

Medical termination of pregnancy

- Can be performed at any gestation.
- If ≥ 21 weeks' gestation feticide is performed first with intracardiac potassium chloride by a fetal medicine expert.
- Oral mifepristone followed 36 hours later with a prostaglandin (misoprostol or gemprost).
- Results in vaginal delivery.
- Timing of delivery is unpredictable.
- Risks of bleeding, retained products of conception.
- Requires adequate analgesia.

Surgical termination of pregnancy

- Can be performed by suction or dilatation and evacuation up to 24 weeks' gestation, although rarely performed after 18 weeks gestation.
- May require cervical priming with a prostaglandin.
- Procedure involves cervical dilatation.
- Risks include uterine perforation, infection, bleeding.
- Requires skilled operators.
- Usually performed under general anaesthesia but can be performed with regional anaesthesia or sedation.

Specific cardiac conditions

Hypertension

- Progestogen-only contraceptives and the copper IUD do not increase blood pressure or cardiovascular events and are safe to use.
- Combined oral contraceptive pills:
  - small risk of developing hypertension (relative risk 1.8) especially if used method for > 5 years (risk decreases when stopped)
  - small elevation in BP in mild hypertensives.

Ischaemic heart disease (IHD)

- Absolute risk of IHD is very small in women of reproductive age even if they have known risk factors.
- Progesterone-only contraceptives (see Table 23.4):
  - no increase in risk of myocardial infarction
  - LNG-IUS safest–better lipid profile (increased HDL levels)
  - use injectable progestogens, POP and Implanon® with caution (moderately unfavourable alterations in lipid metabolism particularly with injectables)
- Combined hormonal contraception are contraindicated:
  - dose-related increase in MI in users taking between 30–50 μg oestradiol (adjusted odds ratio 2.5)
  - risk of MI is not increased in users of 20 μg oestradiol preparations, users of 3rd generation COC and past users of COC
  - risks of MI is further increased by 9–10 fold if smoke, hypertension, or hypercholesterolaemia
- Copper IUD is safe.

Pulmonary hypertension

- Maternal mortality rates up to 40%.
- Use the most efficaceous non-thrombogenic contraceptives: progestogen-only are contraceptively ideal.
- Implanon® : most suitable method increase dose if on bosentan
- Cerazette® slightly less efficaceous increase dose if on bosentan
- Coil insertion (copper or LNG-IUS) causes vasovagal episode in ≥1.2% due to cervical dilatation (LNG-IUS > copper IUD):
  - bradycardias are poorly tolerated: and can lead to circulatory collapse
  - if coil insertion is necessary, insert in hospital with an anaesthetist present and atropine available
- Injectable progestogens are unsuitable if patient is on warfarin.
- Combined hormonal contraceptives contraindicated (thrombotic risk).
- Female sterilisation may be performed without instrumenting the uterus.
- Vasectomy is not recommended as the male usually outlives his partner.

Obstetric care for the non-obstetrician

Terminology

- Primiparous ("primip"): first pregnancy.
- Multiparous ("multip"): ≥1 previous delivery ≥ 24 weeks.
- Gestation is calculated from the last menstrual period (LMP).
- Term: 37–42 weeks' gestation.
- Pre-term: < 37 weeks.
- Estimated date of delivery (EDD): 40 weeks.
- Viability: ≥ 24 weeks (gestation at which if delivered, fetus has a chance of survival: see Table 22.5).
- Multiple pregnancies: twins/triplet or higher order pregnancies.

Antenatal care

The aim of antenatal care is:
- to identify women who require specialist support
- identify uncomplicated pregnancies
- inform pregnant women about pregnancy, childhood and parenting
- mother carries her notes (hand-held notes).

Booking visit

Before 12 weeks' gestation (12/40). Allows:
- identification of risk factors (see Table 24.1)
- allocation of low risk women to midwifery care with GP input (shared care), and high risk women to obstetric care in a hospital environment (obstetric care)
- provision of one to one midwifery support for vulnerable women (e.g. domestic violence, teenagers, single mothers, socially deprived)
- provision of advise to women on:
  - lifestyle issues and diet
  - taking folic acid 0.4 mg until 12 weeks' gestation to prevent neural tube defects (NTD)
  - antenatal classes
  - avoiding contact sports and scuba diving
  - domestic violence
- Screening for maternal risk factors (Table 24.2).
  - Anaemia—iron deficiency: supplement with ferrous sulphate.
  - Atypical blood group antibodies.
  - Rhesus negative: require anti-D at routinely at 28 and 34 weeks and following sensitizing events (e.g. antepartum haemorrhage, amniocentesis) to prevent rhesus alloimmunisation (occurs if carrying a fetus that is rhesus positive).
  - Haemoglobinopathies—e.g. if sickle cell trait or β-thalassaemia trait, need partner testing.
  - Infections—HIV, rubella, syphilis, hepatitis B, UTI.

Table 24.1 Maternal risk factors

Related to mother	Related to previous pregnancy
Age ≤ 18 years or ≥ 40 years	Previous caesarean section
BMI ≤ 17 or ≥ 35	Previous Group B streptococcus
Pre-existing medical disease, e.g. hypertension, diabetes, cardiac, respiratory, renal, endocrine, neurological, psychiatric, connective tissue and haematological diseases, cancer, HIV	Previous pregnancy related disease, e.g. pre-eclampsia, eclampsia, gestational diabetes, obstetric cholestasis, postnatal depression
Family history of genetic disorder	Recurrent miscarriages (≥3)
Lack of social support	Previous midtrimester loss
Domestic violence	Previous pre-term labour
Group B streptococcus carriage	Previous stillbirth or neonatal death
	Previous baby with a congenital abnormality
	Previous baby with intrauterine growth restriction (IUGR)
	Previous baby with macrosomia

Table 24.2 Maternal tests done at booking visit

Bloods	Urine tests	Clinical
FBC	Urine dipstick	Blood pressure
Blood group and rhesus status	MSU	height
Haemoglobin electrophoresis		weight
Rubella IgG		calculation of BMI
Hepatitis B surface Ag		
VDRL/TPHA		
HIV IgM/IgG		

Fetal screening

Aim
- Identification of singleton or multiple pregnancies.
- Confirming viability.
- Confirming gestation.
- Ascertaining risk of Down's syndrome (Trisomy 21).

Screening for Down's syndrome (see Table 24.3)
- Maternal age and.
- Ultrasound for nuchal translucency (NT) and/or.
- Maternal serum biochemistry.

Table 24.3 Different methods of screening for Down's syndrome

Method	NT	11–14 wks bloods*	15–20 wks bloods**	Detection rate	False positive rate
NT	✓			77%	5%
Combined	✓	✓		82–87%	5%
Triple test			hCG, AFP, uE3	69%	5%
Quadruple test			✓ + hCG	81%	7%
Serum integrated		✓	✓	85–88%	5%
Integrated	✓	✓	✓	95%	5%

NT = nuchal translucency   * hCG + PAPP-A   **AFP, uE3, inhibin A

Definitive testing for Down's syndrome or other chromosomal abnormalities:
- chorionic villous sampling (CVS) 11–14 weeks' gestation
- amniocentesis ≥ 15 weeks' gestation
- both carry 1% additional risk of miscarriage.

Screening for congenital malformations
- Major structural anomalies are present in 3% at 20 weeks.
- Anomaly USS 18–20 weeks' gestation: for structural abnormalities.
- Fetal echocardiogram approx 16–23 weeks: for cardiac abnormalities in women with congenital heart disease.

Subsequent visits
- Screen for maternal and fetal wellbeing.
- At each visit the following are checked:
  - maternal BP   } at each visit
  - urine dipstick for proteinuria and glycosuria

- symphisio-fundal height: marker of fetal growth
- fetal viability (maternal perception of fetal movements or auscultation of fetal heart rate)
- fetal lie (i.e. longitudinal/transverse/oblique)
- fetal presentation (i.e. cephalic/breech)
- degree of engagement of fetal presenting part in pelvis.

at each visit ≥ 25 weeks

Table 24.4 Antenatal care schedule

Gestation (weeks)	Specific action
≤ 12	Booking visit: identify risk factors, pregnancy advise, screening tests fetal ultrasound scan
16	Obtain results of screening tests, antenatal classes information
	Appropriate pattern of care scheduled
18–20	Anomaly scan: check fetal viability, growth, fetal anomalies, amniotic fluid volume, placental localisation
28	FBC and atypical red cell antibodies antibodies checked
	Anti D if Rhesus negative
	Glucose tolerance test (GTT) if high risk for gestational diabetes
34	Anti D if Rhesus negative
36	Check fetal presentation- if breech discuss external cephalic version
38	
41	Plans made for induction of labour (IOL)
	Vaginal examination and membrane sweep offered
	Labour induced in low risk women between 41–42 weeks

Additional visits at 25 and 32 weeks if primiparous.

Delivery

Induction of labour

- The cervix is normally 4 cm long, positioned posteriorly and has a firm consistency.
- The cervix needs to become thin (effaced), soft, positioned anteriorly, and dilated
- Cervical softening and thinning (effacement) is induced with vaginal prostaglandin PGE_1 (tablets/gel/long acting agent) called: "prostin/propess".
- Once effaced and 1–2 cm dilated ("favourable"), the membranes are broken (artificial rupture of membranes—ARM).
- Syntocinon (similar to oxytocin) is administered i.v. to stimulate uterine contractions.

Mode of delivery

Vaginal delivery

- First stage of labour: is up to 10 cm cervical dilatation:
  - latent phase of labour is until 3 cm dilatation (variable duration)
  - active phase of labour >3 cm dilatation: cervix dilates approx 1 cm/hour
- Second stage of labour: 10 cm (full dilatation) to delivery of the baby:
  - passive—allows descent of fetal head
  - active (pushing)—allows delivery of baby.
- Third stage of labour is: delivery of the placenta.
- Vaginal delivery has overall less complications than caesarean section.
- Specific considerations in cardiac patients.
  - Effective analgesia in labour to prevent pain induced tachycardia
  - Deliver sitting upright with feet supported.

Assisted vaginal delivery

An instrument (ventouse/forceps) is used to deliver the baby at full dilatation due to: prolonged second stage; fetal distress; if mother has been advised not to push.

Caesarean section (CS)

- Elective—planned to suit.
- Emergency:
  - before onset of labour if complications occur compromising the mother or baby and she is not suitable for induction of labour
  - during labour.
- Maternal risks of CS include haemorrhage, infection, visceral damage, thromboembolism, and risks in future pregnancies of placenta praevia and scar dehiscence or rupture.
- Fetal risk if pre-labour caesarean section of admission to special care baby unit for transient tachypnoea of newborn (TTN) or respiratory distress syndrome (RDS).

Table 24.5 Serious morbidity with caesarean sections

	Risk	Frequency
Maternal	Hysterectomy	0.7–0.8%???
	Further surgery	0.5%
	Bladder injury	0.1%
	Death	1/12,000
Fetal	Lacerations	2%
	Admission to NICU 37 weeks 38 weeks 39 weeks	0.4–0.8% 0.4% 0.4%
Future pregnancies	Placenta praevia/accreta	0.4–0.8%
	Scar dehiscence/rupture	0.4%
	Stillbirth	0.4%

NICU = neonatal intensive care unit

Obstetric indications for Caesarean section

- Malpresentation, e.g. transverse lie or breech
- Placenta praevia
- Cervical fibroid
- Failure to progress in first stage labour
- Fetal distress
- Maternal complications, e.g. severe bleeding
- Failed instrumental delivery.

Cardiac indications for Caesarean section

- Severe left ventricular impairment
- Dilated aortic root.

Pain relief in labour

- Water-lying in warm water in a bath or birthing pool.
- Transcutaneous electrical nerve stimulation (TENS).
- Inhaled entonox: nitrous oxide (50%) and oxygen (50%).
- Narcotics, e.g. diamorphine, patient controlled fentanyl.
- Regional analgesia, e.g epidural, combined spinal epidural, spinal.

Postnatal

Post-partum haemorrhage (PPH)
- Blood loss > 500ml within 24 hours of delivery.
- Identify cause of bleeding, resuscitate and treat cause (see Table 24.6).

Table 24.6 Causes of PPH

Main causes	Treatment
Retained placenta (partial/ complete)	Manual removal of placenta
Uterine atony	Medical: using uterotonics: ergometrine, syntocinon infusion, carbeprost (prostaglandin $PGF_{2\alpha}$), misoprostol
	Surgical: intrauterine balloon, Brace suture, internal iliac artery ligation, uterine artery embolization, hysterectomy
Perineal tears	Repair

Breast feeding
- Encouraged in all patients unless clinically significant concentrations of harmful drug in breast milk.
- Most drugs have negligible concentrations in breast milk and are safe in breast feeding.
- ACE inhibitors and beta blockers are not a contraindication to breast feeding.

Contraception
See Chapter 23.

Assisted reproduction techniques and surrogacy

Infertility

- This is defined as the inability to conceive naturally.
- It is common affecting 1:6 couples.
- Main causes: anovulation, tubal factor (blocked fallopian tubes), male factor (reduced number +/− defective sperm), unexplained.

Treatments available

- In-utero insemination (IUI)—insertion of partner's or donor sperm directly into uterus through the cervix.
- Ovulation induction—clomiphene citrate (Clomid) is given between D2–D6 of the menstrual cycle. It stimulates the ovaries to develop follicles containing eggs.
  Clomid:
  - is a strong antioestrogen and weak oestrogen
  - increases gonadotrophin releasing hormone (GnRH) secretion
  - causes multiple follicles containing eggs to develop
  - risk of ovarian hyperstimulation syndrome (OHSS) small (see page 320)
  - risk of multiple pregnancy 5–10%.
- Assisted reproduction techniques (ART)—different types of artificial and partially artificial means to become pregnant (see p.316).

Considerations prior to treatment

- If pregnancy is not advised on medical grounds, e.g. pulmonary hypertension, severe LV dysfunction DO NOT offer any form of infertility treatment.
- Will drugs used in treatment affect the cardiac condition?
  - Drugs used mimic effects of menstrual cycle.
  - Some fertility specialists use unconventional drugs, e.g. LMWH, intravenous immunoglobulin (IVIG), prednisolone. These do not impact on cardiac disease generally.
- Will procedures required for treatments affect the cardiac condition? See Figure 25.1.
  - OHSS causes severe fluid shifts.
  - Egg collection is painful—ensure adequate analgesia to prevent tachycardia.
  - cervical dilatation with instrumentation can cause a vagal induced bradycardia.

Assisted reproduction techniques (ART)

In-vitro fertilisation (IVF)

A general term describing the fertilisation of an egg and sperm in the laboratory.

Involves various stages (see Figure 25.1):

1. *Superovulation*—normal cycle downregulated with GnRH analogues, or GnRH antagonists. Ovaries stimulated with injections of FSH → development of multiple follicles containing eggs. Ovulation is timed with injection of agents mimicking LH surge, e.g hCG (human chorionic gonadotrophin) or hMG (human menopausal gonadotrophin)
2. *Egg collection*—in a theatre setting. Eggs collected via a needle inserted through the vaginal wall into the pelvis under transvaginal ultrasound guidance. Fluid containing individual eggs aspirated from follicles and given to embryologist. Painful procedure requiring analgesia and i.v. sedation
3. *Sperm collection*—ejaculated sample of partner's or donor sperm → separation of normal motile sperm
4. *Fertilisation*—each egg is mixed with sperm in a petri dish.
5. *Embryo culture*—after fertilisation, embryos develop over 2–5 days. The best embryos are selected and either implanted immediately (fresh cycle) or frozen for use at a later date (cryopreserved)
6. *Embryo transfer*—placement of embryo(s) through cervix into the uterus. Involves manipulation and dilatation of the cervix which can result in a vagally induced bradycardia. Success rates are 28–35%.

Intra-cytoplasmic sperm insemination (ICSI)

As for IVF except one sperm is injected directly into one egg with a microneedle to achieve fertilisation. This method is used in instances of male factor infertililty. Sperm is collected either via ejaculation with subsequent sperm sorting to identify active healthy sperm, or collected directly from the testis or epidydimus. 35% success rates. ICSI is more expensive than IVF.

Gamete intrafallopian transfer (GIFT)

Eggs are collected laparoscopically then injected surgically with sperm into the fallopian tubes where fertilisation occurs. Low success rate.

Zygote intrafallopian transfer (ZIFT)

Similar to GIFT, but fertilisation occurs first *in vitro* and then the zygote is injected into a fallopian tube. Low success rate.

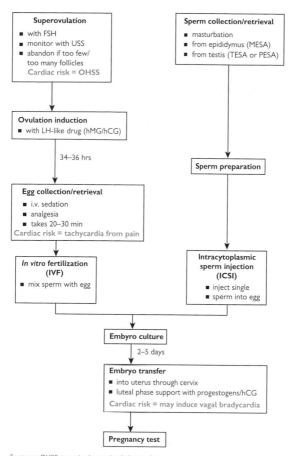

Footnote: OHSS = ovarian hyperstimulation syndrome

Fig. 25.1 Steps used for *in-vitro* fertilization and intracytoplasmic sperm injection.

Risks of ART

Maternal
- Multiple pregnancy.
- Ovarian hyperstimulation syndrome (OHSS).
- Infection (including pelvic abscess: rare).
- Bleeding at egg collection (rare).
- Increased risk of pre-eclampsia, particularly with egg donation.

Fetal
- Slight increase in birth defects with ART (OR 1.3 major birth defects compared to naturally conceived children matched for maternal age).
- Low birth weight.
- Preterm birth.

Ovarian hyperstimulation syndrome (OHSS)

Systemic disease resulting from vasoactive products released from hyper-stimulated ovaries. Leads to:
- enlarged ovaries
- increased capillary permeability + low oncotic pressure → fluid shifts into 3rd space (pleural effusions, ascites, pericardial effusion) → oliguria (intravascular depletion)
- hypercoaguable state due to haemoconcentration → thrombosis
- severity can worsen over time.

Risk factors for developing OHSS
- Multiple follicles develop in ovulation induction or superovulation cycles.
- Age < 30 years.
- Polycystic ovaries.
- Pregnancy in treatment cycle.
- Previous OHSS.

Incidence
- Mild OHSS up to 33% with IVF.
- Severe OHSS 3–8% with IVF.

Clinical
- Abdominal distension and pain.
- Nausea and vomiting.

Treatment
Supportive until spontaneous resolution:
- analgesia with paracetamol/codeine/opiates depending on severity
- admit if severe OHSS: massive ovaries, acute fluid shifts
- critical OHSS requires intensive care admission
- strict fluid balance and daily measurement of weight and abdominal girth
- daily U+E, LFT, albumin, FBC, clotting
- fluid input 2–3L/day
- thromboprophylaxis with LMWH
- human albumin infusion/ 6% hydroxyethylstarch (HES) in severe OHSS
- ascitic and pleural taps may be necessary
- diuretics rarely used.

Complications
- Thrombosis.
- Renal failure.
- Liver failure.
- ARDS.
- Death.

Egg donation

Used by women with:
- premature ovarian failure: no eggs due to surgery, chemotherapy, autoimmune disease
- genetic conditions
- poor quality eggs due to advanced maternal age
- previously unsuccessful IVF cycles.

Surrogacy

Another woman (surrogate mother) has a baby and agrees to give the baby after delivery to the couple with whom an arrangement has been made. The genetics of the baby will depend on the exact arrangement:
- natural conception
- IUI with partner's sperm/ selected donor sperm
- IVF or ICSI with partner's sperm
- IVF using couple's egg and sperm and embryo transfer into uterus of surrogate mother.

Surrogacy is an option if:
- patient's medical condition is so severe that pregnancy is not recommended
- patient has ovaries but no uterus (congenital absence/previous surgical removal)
- patient has no ovaries and no uterus.

Assisted conception and the law in the UK

Human Fertilisation and Embryology Act 1990

Published in response to concerns regarding the creation of human embryos outside the body and their use in treatment and research, and the use of donated gametes and embryos.

Activities prohibited in the act

- Keeping or using an embryo in vitro after the appearance of the primitive streak or 14 days of development, whichever is the earlier.
- Placing a human embryo in a non-human animal.
- Cloning—replacing the nucleus of an embryo with a nucleus from another person/another embryo.
- Altering the genetic structure of any cell while it forms part of an embryo.

Human Fertility and Embryology Authority (HFEA)

- Established in 1991 as a statutory non-departmental public regulator with powers to license and inspect premises conducting assisted conception.
- Accountable to the Secretary of State for Health.
- Publishes and revises regularly its code of practice.
- Keeps register of all treatment cycles and of all children born with ART or with donated eggs/sperm.
- Such children born can request to know if they were born from treatment requiring an HFEA license, and can request to know the identity of donor once they reach age 18 years.

Licenses granted by HFEA

- Treatment license: required for IVF, ICSI, PGD, donation of sperm, eggs and embryos, surrogacy.
- Storage license: cryopreservation.
- Research license: for human embryos in vitro.

Number of embryos that can be transferred

- Age <40 years: 2 ⎱ in the UK
- Age >40 years: 3 ⎰
- Variable numbers elsewhere; some countries have no limits—effects of infertility tourism causes problems in the UK (multiple pregnancies and their consequences).

Implications of the HFEA for practice

- *Consent*—Detailed written consent for exact circumstances of use of gametes required from the provider(s) of those gametes (without the notion of ownership). Includes naming individuals donating and receiving gametes/embryos.
- *Confidentiality*—Criminal sanctions if confidentiality breached. Information about treatment can be passed onto a third party with the patient's written consent.
- *Counselling*—Consent not valid unless counselling by a trained fertility counsellor offered on the implications of taking the proposed steps.
- *Information*—Appropriate information about treatment must be given before proceeding, including current success rates (live birth rate per treatment cycle).
- *Welfare of the child*—A woman shall not be provided with treatment services unless account has been taken of the welfare of any child who may be born as a result of the treatment and of any other child who may be affected by the birth (existing children in the family).

Legal parents of children from donated gametes or surrogacy

Donated sperm

- Woman's husband is the legal father of the child unless:
  - they are judicially separated or
  - he can prove he did not consent to the treatment.
- Woman's male partner whom she has entered into treatment with is the legal father:
  - if she does not have a legal husband or
  - if her legal husband does not consent to treatment.

Donated eggs

- Woman who has received the eggs ("birth mother") is the legal mother and her partner or husband is the legal father.

Surrogacy

- Child needs to be adopted even though genetically derived from one or both parents.
- Birth mother and her partner or husband are legal parents until legal parentage is transferred to the commissioning couple.
- Birth mother and her partner must register birth with their names as parents.
- Surrogacy arrangements between commissioning couple and the surrogate mother are not legally enforceable under UK law.

Obstetric anaesthesia and cardiac disease

Introduction

Although decisions regarding mode and timing of delivery are primarily determined by obstetric and cardiac indications, the anaesthetist has an important role in enabling a safe and optimal outcome for both mother and baby.

Mode of delivery and anaesthetic technique

Vaginal delivery

- *Regional analgesia* describes pain relief provided by neural blockade usually via epidural or combined spinal and epidural (CSE) techniques in labour.
- Modern techniques commonly involve the epidural administration of low-dose mixtures of local anaesthetics and opiates, providing adequate sensory loss with minimum motor blockade ("mobile epidurals").
- An effective labour epidural can be topped up as appropriate if an assisted delivery (forceps, ventouse) or Caesarean section (CS) becomes necessary, AND if time allows.
- In women with cardiac disease aiming for a vaginal delivery, regional analgesia for pain relief in labour provides additional benefits:

Advantages

- The low-dose mixture commonly used avoids haemodynamic compromise and maintains uteroplacental perfusion (**NB** Invasive haemodynamic monitoring may still be necessary—this should be decided on a case-by-case basis).
- Obtunds stress response associated with labour/pushing (decrease in release of catecholamines, avoids tachycardia/hypertension)
- Decreased SVR/afterload.

Contraindications to regional analgesia

- Patient refusal.
- Coagulopathy—including treatment with heparin.

(Regional analgesia in the presence of low dose aspirin therapy is accepted to be safe but clopidogrel is still a contraindication with majority of obstetric anaesthetists)

- Fixed cardiac output.
- Bacteraemia/local sepsis.

Caesarean section

Regional anaesthesia (RA) describes dense neural blockade such as that required for a pain-free operative delivery.

- It is associated with autonomic blockade including cardiac sympathetic blockade, so uncontrolled, rapid-onset regional anaesthesia is especially dangerous in cardiac disease.
- An experienced obstetric anaesthetist can avoid haemodynamic instability using:
  - incremental induction of RA
  - infusion of appropriate vasopressor to control peripheral vasodilation (e.g. phenylephrine)
  - judicious co-load of intravenous fluid.

Advantages of RA for CS
- Avoids risks associated with general anaesthesia.
- Optimal postoperative analgesia.
- Mother may be able to eat and drink immediately postoperatively.
- Birth partner can be present at delivery to support mother.
- Mother awake at time of birth therefore greater chance for bonding.

Contraindications to RA for CS are the same as for regional analgesia in labour.

General anaesthesia (GA) was until relatively recently the preferred anaesthetic technique for CS in women with cardiac disease.

Advantages of GA for CS
- Allows standard therapeutic thromboprophylaxis/anticoagulation to be continued peripartum because no risk of spinal/epidural haematoma.
- It is relatively quick to establish anaesthesia and then deliver baby.
- Haemodynamic stability may be maintained using cardiostable induction of anaesthesia (usually high dose benzodiazepine/opiate mixture, thus minimizing need for usual induction agents such as propofol or thiopentone, which are primarily responsible for hypotension on induction of anaesthesia). Cardiostable induction drugs also attenuate hypertensive response to laryngoscopy and intubation.
- Enables optimal oxygenation of patient (particularly important to avoid hypoxic pulmonary vasoconstriction).
- Enables optimal positioning of patient for surgery, i.e. patient able to be laid flat, which may not be possible with regional.
- Any complications during surgery can be managed quickly.
- May be less stressful for patient (decreased catecholamine release, decreased sympathetic tone).

Disadvantages of GA for CS
- Drugs required for cardiostable induction cross placenta so baby at increased risk of requiring post-partum oxygenation/ventilatory assistance because of neonatal respiratory depression.
- Anaesthetic gases are myocardial depressants but risk of maternal awareness if anaesthesia too light because anaesthetist trying to minimise this effect.
- All pregnant women recognised to be at greater risk of failed intubation and thus aspiration of gastric contents. This would be catastrophic with concomitant cardiac disease.
- Increased risk of blood loss associated with CS under GA.
- Postoperative pain, nausea and vomiting, respiratory depression, thrombosis all more likely after GA than RA.
- Anaesthetized mother unable to see/immediately bond with baby.

Choice of anaesthetic technique

Depends on:
1. Medical needs of the mother.
2. Preference of anaesthetist.
3. Relative importance of all risk factors in individual case.
4. Wishes of mother.

There is no robust evidence to support the use of one technique over the other in pregnant women with cardiac disease, although regional techniques are increasingly being used.

General considerations for the obstetric anaesthetist

Uterotonic agents

Obstetric haemorrhage is poorly tolerated in cardiac disease so adequate uterine contraction after delivery of the placenta is essential. Use of uterotonic agents in severe cardiac disease however, remains controversial.

- **Oxytocin**—usually given as an i.v. bolus dose (5 i.v.) after delivery of the baby. Known to cause decrease in blood pressure due to peripheral vasodilation and decreased cardiac contractility/HR. Slow iv infusion generally accepted to be haemodynamically stable (e.g. author's protocol : 5 iu in 50 ml Nsaline over 20–30 mins). Oxytocin infusions should be administered in minimal volumes of fluid as it has an ADH-like effect and may precipitate fluid overload. *Use with particular caution in conditions which tolerate vasodilation poorly, i.e. PHT, AS, HCM, etc*
- **Ergometrine**—contraindicated in some cardiac disease as increases SVR and can precipitate coronary artery vasospasm. *Avoid particularly in coarctation, pre-eclampsia etc*
- **Carboprost (PGF2$_\alpha$) and misoprostol**—both contraindicated in patients with myocardial ischaemia. In addition, carboprost may cause bronchospasm. Side effects of misoprostol include shivering (increases oxygen consumption) and hyperpyrexia (rare but serious). Use of both agents require further investigation in cardiac disease.

Mechanical manoeuvres may be used as an alternative, or in addition to, pharmacological uterotonic agents. These include:
1. bimanual compression of the uterus
2. compression sutures
3. intra-uterine balloons.

Maternal monitoring

- The level of haemodynamic monitoring required peripartum should be decided on a case-by-case basis.
- Invasive monitoring is not always necessary in women with cardiac disease, but is usually used if Caesarean section is planned.

Autotransfusion

- On delivery of the placenta, there is an autotransfusion of approximately 500 ml of blood from the uteroplacental circulation into the maternal circulation.
- This fluid bolus may not be well tolerated in some cardiac conditions (particularly mitral stenosis).
- The anaesthetist may consider pre-emptive diuresis (e.g. using furosemide) prior to delivery to avoid fluid overload/pulmonary oedema.

Postoperative care (for CS)

- Depending on the patient condition and the facilities available, postoperative care may necessitate transfer to an intensive care or coronary care unit.
- This in turn will limit access of mother to baby and to midwives.
- It is therefore preferable, if safe and staffing/facilities allow, for mother to be monitored on a High Dependency Unit on Delivery Suite.

Conclusion

The multidisciplinary team should include an obstetric anaesthetist and all members of the team must liaise closely to formulate a definitive anaesthetic management plan for delivery. Anaesthetic considerations include:

- Mode of delivery
- Anaesthetic technique
- Management of third stage
- Monitoring required
- Fluid balance including autotransfusion
- Anaesthetic management in event of obstetric/medical complications, e.g. haemorrhage, arrhythmia
- Postoperative care.

Index